D0794121

Transcultural Dimensions in Medical Ethics

Edited by

EDMUND PELLEGRINO
PATRICIA MAZZARELLA
PIETRO CORSI

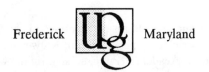

Frederick   Maryland

University Publishing Group, Inc.
Frederick Maryland, 21701

Copyright 1992 by University Publishing Group. All rights reserved
Printed in the United States of America
ISBN 1-55572-015-3

"American Moralism and the Origin of Bioethics in the United States," by
Albert R. Jonsen, is reprinted by permission of Kluwer Academic Publishers.
Copyright 1991 Kluwer Academic Publishers. Originally published in *The
Journal of Medicine and Philosophy* 16, no. 1 (February 1991): 113-30.

Acknowledgments

We wish to thank Fidia Research Foundation, which co-sponsored with Georgetown University the Transcultural Dimensions in Medical Ethics Symposium held at the National Academy of Sciences in Washington, DC, on 26 and 27 April 1990.

The Editors

Contributors

Zbigniew Bankowski, MD, is Secretary-General of the Council for International Organizations of Medical Sciences (CIOMS), World Health Organization, Geneva, Switzerland.

Pietro Corsi, DPhil, is Scientific Secretary, Fidia Research Foundation, Florence.

Attajinda Deepadung is a member of the Faculty of Social Science and Humanities, in the Department of Humanities, Faculty of Social Science and Humanities, Mahidol University, Nakhonprathom, Thailand.

Academician **Ivan T. Frolov** is Chairman of the Scientific Council for Philosophical and Social Problems of Science and Technology; and a Professor at Moscow State University.

Hassan Hathout, MD, PhD, FRCSE, FRCOG, FACS, is a member of the staff of the Islamic Organization of Medical Sciences, Pasadena, California.

Albert R. Johnson, PhD, is Professor of Ethics in Medicine and Chairman of the Department of Medical History and Ethics, School of Medicine, University of Washington, Seattle.

José Alberto Mainetti, MD, is a member of the faculty at the Instituto de Humanidades Médicas y Centro de Bioética, Centro Oncologico de Excelincia de Gonnet, Gonnet, Argentina.

Enrico Chiavacci, PhD, is the Director of the Department of Ethics at the Theological Institute of Florence (Studio Teologico Fiorentino).

C.M. Francis, MD, is Director of St. Martha's Hospital, Bangalore, India.

Shimon Glick, MD, is Gussie Krupp Professor of Internal Medicine at the University Faculty of Health Sciences, Ben Gurion University of the Negev, Beer Sheva, Israel.

Rihito Kimura, JD, is Director of International Bioethics Programs at the Kennedy Institute of Ethics, Georgetown University, Washington, DC; and Professor of Bioethics and Law at the School of Human Sciences, Wasena University, Tokyo.

Patricia Mazzarella, MA, is an Instructor of Bioethics and Philosophy; and a Doctoral Candidate at Georgetown University, Washington, DC.

Robert F. Murray Jr., MD, FACP, is Professor of Pediatrics, Medicine, and Genetics at Howard University College of Medicine, Washington, DC.

Edmund D. Pellegrino, MD, is John Carroll Professor of Medicine and Medical Ethics; Director of the Georgetown University Center for the Advanced Study of Ethics; and Director of the Center for Clinical Bioethics, Washington, DC.

Ren-Zong Qiu is Professor of Bioethics at the Institute of Philosophy, Chinese Academy of Social Sciences, Beijing; and Visiting Professor of Medical Ethics, in the Department of Philosophy, University of Wisconsin-Madison.

B.O. Osuntokun, PhD, MD, DSc (London), FRCP (London), FMCP (Nigeria), is a Professor of Medicine (Neurology) at the Department of Medicine, University of Ibadan, Ibadan, Nigeria; and Visiting Professor (Neurology) at the Department of Psychiatry, Indiana University School of Medicine, Indianapolis.

Contents

1

Introduction

There may be a certain hubris in attempting a transcultural dialogue in medical ethics. What thought patterns can we share as ideas when that we speak from such diverse medical, socio-cultural, genetic, historical, religious, and political frames of reference? The variables are significant and the task of understanding each other appears formidable when viewed from the perspective of our unique special concerns.

Beyond hubris, and beyond the amazement we experience when we consider the gestalt of our efforts from its pluralistic perspective, there is a humble acknowledgement of the possibility of a shift in the gestalt. With time and effort, the dialogue appears to be shaped by the frames of reference of a global community. And the goal, often thought only to be conflict resolution through the development of a method or policy arising out of compromise, becomes the discovery of common values which might guide our thinking as members of this widest possible community. The papers presented in this volume and the subsequent dialogue engendered has been one early effort to begin a frame of reference focussing on the expressed needs, common values, and consequently the medical, research, and related policy goals of the world community.

The term "transcultural dimensions" was carefully chosen. A dimension is that which communicates the nature and scope of units related in some way. Each of the invited authors has contributed an explication of one set of socio-cultural and often religious values as they are interpreted when evaluating the high-priority clinical and research questions of his country. And each offered a consideration of the ways in which these uniquely situated questions might relate to similar issues in other countries or systems of medicine. It is a beginning, one which is based on the recognition that, as Attajinda Deepadung pointed out in his paper, disease is a cultural universal.

We have organized the contributions in a geographical fashion, from west to east and north to south. If we look more closely at the nature and scope of the papers, we see that each value system presented is given in a context of theoretical, applicational, and historical analysis. The authors represent developed and developing countries with traditions rooted in Western, Eastern, African, African-American, Latin-American, Marxist, Christian, Jewish, and Islamic belief systems. The influence of each set of values on the others has brought about a flux in the practiced morality of all. The attempts to articulate this confluence have been the focal points of each contribution.

Albert Jonsen provides a historical and theoretical analysis of the moral tradition within the United States as it has been exhibited in bioethics. He proposes that American culture's matrix morality is American moralism rooted in religious fundamentalism. Based on tenets expressed in Jansenism, Puritanism, and Calvinism, this morality affirms personal liberty and social cohesion, belief in clear, unambiguous principles, and a view of the world as composed of antithetical categories needing boundary systems of control. These boundary systems are provided by unambiguous moral commandments which can be known by a pure will or "heart." There is no room in this system for real paradox. Kierkegaardian moral conflict is only apparent and casuistry, the technique of moral analysis of particular cases, is unacceptable. The principles of this belief system, Professor Jonsen notes, are thought to be grasped by common sense. They do not allow for real exceptions and have a tendency to lump together complex moral issues. It is assumed that if these principles are observed, the good of the community will follow.

Contemporary bioethics has responded to the many questions which led to moral ambiguity by focusing on developing clarity of method. When the task of bioethics passed from representatives of fundamentalist belief systems into the hands of academics and intellectuals, clarity of principle and moral certitude was no longer a respectable stance. Proponents of logical positivism, pragmatism, utilitarianism, and existentialism exercised a significant influence on the discipline. In response to the presentation of a medical-ethical dilemma, probabilistic opinions were sought. It became important to articulate a range of options which could be supported on the strength of rational argument and the logic supporting it.

Professor Jonsen concludes that there are two aspects to the task of addressing medical moral issues in the United States. One is the sociological task of description in which the problem is described as fully and as accurately as possible from the classical American perspective of fundamental moralism. The second is to apply the intellectual techniques of analysis known as ethics. The second has been done well, the first only fitfully and poorly. He proposes that a sociological analysis of the moral dimension, such as that done by Robert Bellah in *Habits of the Heart*, might bring some insight into medical moral problems. Then the dilemmas which are currently relegated to "apparently irreconcilable differences," and which are so often ascribed to "political differences," might be more clearly understood and analyzed.

Robert Murray presents the ethical values of African-Americans, contrasting them with those of Euro-Americans. Reviewing major efforts to identify ethical perspectives in American minority groups, he notes that self-determination has been the theme running throughout the conferences and study projects. Of nearly equal importance were privacy, confidentiality, informed consent, and access to health care. Dr. Murray notes that a long history of suffering, dehumanization, and deprivation has led to an emphasis among African-Americans on a desire to satisfy needs immediately and to seek rapid relief of suffering. As a result there is a "focus on living *carpe diem* and not postponing gratification" which is "a way for people in distress to maintain hope, especially when they live in conditions from which there seems to be no escape. They don't set long-term goals and don't adopt an ethical stance that involves delayed gratification."

There is some conflict in application of the principles most highly valued, particularly that of justice. Allegiance to the group and sharing of resources which is an inheritance from black African roots cannot be reconciled with an emotional commitment to a capitalist ethic. As a result perceived values shift to a more personal level with security/survival ranking first. Others, in order of importance, are power/self-determination, truth-telling, and justice. The most significant bioethical issue for African-Americans reflects their most pressing need--access to and quality of health care.

José Mainetti considers bioethics to be a culture of civil morality as well as an academic, consultative, and policymaking discipline. Outlining the Latin-American perspective on bioethics as it has developed in Argentina, he presents an overview of the conceptual and institutional process as it has evolved over the past twenty years from both academic and everyday experience.

The observations arising from this analysis show a new and unique perspective in Argentina, one which reflects the transcultural shapings that are a result of the influence of Western bioethics in a cultural context that is not its own. The model which has evolved is traditional and paternalistic rather than libertarian. It is opposed to any notion of patient autonomy and is not a legal or judicial endeavor. Dr. Mainetti proposes that the introduction of a rights-based medical ethics arising from the notion of patient autonomy "presumes an increasingly conflictive set of relations between patient, physician, and society." Medical authority is not yet challenged in Argentina and a technicalization of life processes has not yet occurred.

Norms in Argentina take into account the good of the community, and individual choice is not the only basis of medical decisionmaking. This model of bioethics attempts to balance the individual good with the common good in ways that countries focussing on the implementation of autonomy have not been able to do. Dr. Mainetti proposes that this is best done as a consultative and policymaking discipline.

ELABE, the Latin American School of Bioethics of the Mainetti Foundation, is an educational project with the goal of examining bioethical issues and their consequent influence on cultural norms and public policy. Within this context, the goal of the center is to prepare bioethicists to establish programs in their own countries and to serve as a center for cultural and scientific exchange. Dr. Mainetti has coined the term "hygeinomia" to express his view that bioethics ought to be, rather than a synthesis of liberal ethics and technological processes, a synthesis of authentic health and common morality.

Shimon Glick describes the Jewish perspective as a polychromatic picture of the unique amalgam of religion and nationhood which is Judaism. Even though there is a wide temporal, geographic, and philosophic diversity in Judaism, an identifiable cultural core can be extracted. This core expresses the beliefs that human beings have the ultimate responsibility for their own actions and the consequences of those actions, that the world is in motion toward eventual perfection and redemption, that the world will eventually become a fitting environment for the human being, and that human dignity, peace, and social justice will reign in the messianic age.

Human beings have a responsibility to improve both self and society so that we may eliminate strife, suffering, injustice, and ultimately even death. Jewish tradition requires the physician, as well as the non-physician, to render care to someone in distress. This positive obligation is extended to self, meaning that one is required to seek medical care when ill.

Life has an absolutely intrinsic value since it is seen as G-d's creation over which humans are the stewards. Casual contraception, abortion (except to save the life of the mother), infanticide, non-treatment of handicapped newborns, and active euthanasia are all proscribed by Judaism. There is a great respect for the aged and any cost/benefit considerations leading to discrimination are seen to be a fundamental downgrading of the respect for life.

All of life is respected in the Jewish tradition, but there is a hierarchy in which the lower forms serve the higher. Humans are to control nature and use it creatively and constructively. Hunting and activities such as cockfighting are forbidden, but medical research conducted under humane conditions is considered laudable. Medical research contributes to the preservation of life and is a response to the religious command to explore the wonders of nature. Research and medical practices have some limits, however. The integrity of one's family line is valued highly, so germ line therapy with its unknown consequences (as well as surrogate motherhood and non-homologous IVF) is not looked upon favorably.

Respect for life extends to respect for the dead. Burial of the intact body must be done as quickly and respectfully as possible. Autopsies are to be done immediately and only for good reason. There is a great reluctance to allow this and it is unthinkable to allow dissection of unclaimed bodies of the poor. These would have the highest priority for respectful burial by the community.

Jewish tradition is incorporated in the Talmud which has, throughout the ages, addressed a multitude of ethical dilemmas. It is "an elaborate legal and ethical corpus based on eternal values." Since questioning is highly valued in Judaism, the answers to ethical dilemmas are often left open, and such a state of uncertainty is accepted with equanimity.

Hassan Hathout provided a general outline and history of Islam, including the tenets of faith, principles, and Islamic Code of Medical Ethics issued by the Islamic Organization of Medical Sciences in 1981. In order to set Islamic bioethics in context, Dr. Hathout established these tenets, principles, and code in relation to Islam's predecessors, Judaism and Christianity.

Basic tenets of faith are that every human being is born in purity and is responsible for his or her own deeds. Human beings are God's "vice-regents on earth" and have been entrusted with the prescribed plan of the Creator. Human freedom is emphasized as well as responsibility for its proper use.

There is no church in Islam, so separation of church and state is not an issue. The Shari'a, a total system of Islamic law in four principle sources, is the comprehensive framework of regulation of human activities. In the Quran, the Tradition of the Prophet, the Universal Consensus of Scholars, and Analogy (which comprise the Shari'a), creed and belief rulings are fixed while those relating to human relationships allow flexibility based on circumstances. The Islamic basis for bioethics lies in the understanding that human thinking must devise new rulings for new situations as long as there is no conflict with the spirit of the religion or trespassing outside the goals of the Shari'a.

Satisfaction of human needs is the goal of the rulings of the Shari'a. There are indispensable needs such as preservation of body, preservation of mind, religion, ownership, and honor. Ordinary needs are covered by commercial and civil laws. Complementary needs are those which improve life. The role of mankind is to enhance life so that human needs may be met.

Ivan Frolov's contribution traces the history of genetic thought in the Soviet Union, specifically as it took shape with formal organization in 1920 of the Russian Eugenic Society in Moscow under the chairmanship of Koltsoz. He notes that prior to current advances in technology, programs within the Soviet Union were concerned mainly with solving strictly scientific problems. Now, however, it is necessary to address the question of whether it is acceptable to change human nature through eugenics. Reasoning from the premise that it is scientifically unsound to propose neo-eugenic projects which might create the "ideal man," Professor Frolov maintains that, even if possible, such projects would play a reactionary social role. The application of such programs, he states, would produce a genetic catastrophe. Based on respect for human freedom and uniqueness, he encourages further development of the social aspects of genetic-anthropological research and their humanistic orientation. Such an approach is desirable because it precludes scientistic and manipulative approaches to human beings which limit their personal freedom.

Enrico Chiavacci presents an overall view of bioethics which addresses the problem of pluralism in varying ethical contexts and cultures. He proposes that ethics is a process of studying and discovering the common aim or "ideal of solidarity" shared by developed and developing countries alike. All are members of the complex system which is the human family. If we accept this complexity and learn to live with it, we also accept the paradox of attempting to achieve a consensus of ethical guidelines while preserving the cultural identities of members of this family.

The foundation for cooperation in the search for the common good and common goals lies in the realization that happiness is a result of self-giving rather than self-realization. The good life is found in the implementation of the rights of solidarity as found in Europe and which contrasts with the rights of liberty as dominant in the United States. The rights of solidarity are based on the notion that the community has a positive obligation to help individuals develop and realize themselves, that it cannot interfere with free choice, and that this free choice is limited by the needs and choices of others. This contrasts with the notion that rights are based only on an individual's unrestricted free choices. In such a liberty-based ethic, the community has no positive obligation other than to provide as few restrictions as possible.

This notion of morality, based on rights of solidarity, places a responsibility on the physician to provide for the complete well-being of patients, not just to treat and attempt to cure the disease processes. Physicians are first, to do no harm. But this must be practiced in a context of loyalty to the patient that goes beyond a business relationship to one which expresses agapic love and respect for him or her as a complete human being within community. This may be accomplished by honoring a covenant in which both patient and physician have choices based on intrinsically valuable principles. There are some boundaries to such a covenant, however, and these may be evident when the values of one conflict with the other.

Addressing the question of distributive justice, Professor Chiavacci notes that basic medical needs are not yet satisfied for a large majority of today's human family. The accepted notion that a doctor has an ethical responsibility to an individual patient ought to be widened to a framework in which doctors, researchers, and institutions ought to consider their ethical responsibilities at a global level.

In order to act on these responsibilities, it is necessary to set goals which take into account the problems of hunger in the world and the threat of nuclear war with its concomitant problem of the arms race. To pursue one's own happiness is not possible, Professor Chiavacci maintains, unless the well-being of all of humanity is improving. One's own happiness depends on this improvement, just as the well-being of a family member depends on the good health of the family as a whole.

B.O. Osuntokun emphasizes that the primary health care issue for developing countries is justice and equity in resource allocation and distribution of health care resources. Pointing out that WHO has accepted primary health care as the cornerstone of national health care systems, he states that this essential need is not being met in sub-Saharan Africa.

In the last decade, the health of the population in sub-Saharan Africa has deteriorated due to widespread poverty and a poor economy which supports neither a research infrastructure nor control of ethical issues. There continues to be lack of adequate access to the modern necessities of life--clean water supply, education, hygienic housing facilities, and health care services. In many of the countries, as much as eighty percent of the population has no access to health care.

Other ethical issues concern research that is done in sub-Saharan Africa, reproductive health, and organ transplantation. He calls to question the practices of obtaining "informed consent" for research from community leaders rather than individuals, of exclusion criteria based on age or difficulty in enrolling, of parallel tracks (giving patients not included in controlled drug trials unapproved drugs), and of the withholding of data from public health authorities in the country in which the research was done. He calls for minimal ethical standards which may be such as those specified by CIOMS with some cultural modifications as needed.

The most important value to be considered is respect for human dignity. This non-negotiable basis for ethical treatment may involve the establishment of a national medical ethics commission and of regional, local, and institutional ethics committees. Dr. Osuntokun states that ethical principles are unchanging, while the guidelines arising from these basic statements of value should by dynamic and periodically reviewed.

Since people in developing countries are becoming increasingly better educated, and political emancipation is changing the perception of the role of the individual in society and the community, new issues continue to arise which must be addressed. Resolution depends on the establishment of well-administered legal and policymaking institutions.

Rihito Kimura stresses that the notion of harmony as achieved through sharing is of primary importance in Japanese bioethics. In Japanese tradition, the egoistic self must be suppressed so that the sharing of *kyokan* (feeling togetherness) as *ningen* (human person in a relational context) may take place. This principle addresses the need for people to be dependent on one another in the family, social, economic, and political community. It conflicts, however, with the notion of autonomy which is considered an egocentric idea.

In his contribution, Professor Kimura provides a socio-historical background of Japanese medicine. There has always been a great respect for law, order, authority, and social status which reflects the fact that Japanese mentality is based on a Confucian ethos. Physicians have typically been paternalistic and authoritative, expecting compliance with decisions due to their status in the community.

The younger generation of Japanese is beginning to question this tradition, preferring group decisionmaking and truth concerning diagnosis. Since Japanese society is structured on traditional family values and each person is expected to behave with full sensitivity to the harmony of relationships, decisionmaking may be based on a sense of shared responsibility. This is becoming the case with neonatal care providers at the local, regional, and national levels. The medical team communicates with the family both by speaking to them and by writing notes about the problem, the process of treatment, and their feelings on the situation and possible decisions. They thereby become a cooperative support system and a sensitive part of the decisionmaking process.

In the People's Republic of China, bioethical dilemmas are much the same as those emerging elsewhere in the world. Ethicists, physicians, and the public are concerned with the morality of euthanasia, abortion, in vitro fertilization, and methods of population control as well as with the practice of infanticide and issues related to treatment of the handicapped.

Ren-Zong Qiu addresses the issues raised by these dilemmas from the contemporary Chinese perspective. He discusses them in the context of their background in Chinese history and the current sociocultural influences affecting public opinion and morality as it is developing in practice. In his final section, Professor Qiu considers the ways in which the proposed moral framework is similar and the ways in which it is different, both from the traditional approach and from Western bioethics.

The recorded history of Chinese medicine is at least two thousand years old. Professor Qiu notes that the first code of medical ethics was written by Sun Simiao in the seventh century AD. It arose out of a culture grounded in the Three Teachings: Confucianism, Buddhism, and Taoism, which provided a conceptual framework for the explanation and treatment of disease. Treatment was based on principles and virtues which had as their aim the restoration of harmony within the patient. Such a restoration was, in part, a result of a harmonious relationship between physician and patient who must, in order to achieve this state, continue to work at personal self-cultivation and seek moral transformation.

Chinese medical ethics is a virtue-based morality with a deontological basis. According to this approach, the most important effect of character-building by self-cultivation is compassion. There are many maxims which express unchanging heavenly principles, but these cannot be applied in situations of judgment unless the physician has experienced a moral transformation. Professor Qiu points out that, in the Chinese culture, external constraints such as rules and laws are not the preferred method of bringing about harmony in the person or in relationships. Rather, this balance is ideally achieved through the wisdom of each individual as he or she is transformed by living the Three Teachings.

Living well, or quality of life for both individuals and society as a whole, is a primary value in the People's Republic of China. Along with the belief that humanity begins at birth, this value affects both professional and public moral intuitions on all issues, especially those of euthanasia, abortion, infanticide, and allocation of scarce resources. In recent years, since Marxism with its historicity and social holism has become the dominant ideology, moral decisions have gone in the direction of concern for the community and the future rather than for the individual and the present. Currently, however, Western influences have brought about an increased interest in promoting the individual good. As a result, Professor Qiu concludes, there is a presently a high level of uncertainly both in society and medical ethics, leaving morality in flux.

Attajinda Deepadung emphasizes the conceptual elements that underlie all aspects of traditional Thai medical systems. Presenting an overview of these systems and their interaction with Western systems of medicine, he argues that such traditional methods are integral parts of total cultural patterns which function as effective adaptive strategies to the threats posed by diseases.

Medical behavior cannot be separated from cultural history. We must, then, evaluate Thai traditional medical systems by first identifying the perception within the culture of the causes of illness. It will follow that the commonly accepted adaptive strategies can be seen as a set of rational responses to such a common perception.

Thai traditional medicine is based on the notion that illness is a result of an imbalance or lack of harmony, both within the society itself and in the sick person's relations with others in the society. The result of this causal perception is that treatments are directed to restoration of psychological and social conditions as well as physiological. A healer does not simply treat symptoms. He or she attempts to restore harmony within the patient's entire environmental context. It is for this reason that public healing ceremonies are performed: they provide a powerful psychosocial support dimension.

This system, as Professor Deepadung points out, has both strengths and weaknesses. The psychotherapeutic effects include emotional catharsis and relief from the burden of guilt-producing experiences (such as those which have brought harm to others in one's community). In addition, support systems are coordinated because healing practices require the presence of family and community members. Another strength is the herbal pharmacopeia which uses medications that alone or in traditional combinations do not have the serious side effects of Western medicines.

The primary weakness of this approach to healing is that its practitioners are generally lacking in basic knowledge of anatomy, physiology, and pathology. Since there are no systematic methods of treatment, teaching is inconsistent and sometimes vague. It is difficult to relate the traditional system to the disease model of medicine, so the results of research within the latter model cannot be used.

As in other countries in which traditional medicine is important, a new school has been developed in Thailand to bring together the traditional and the Western systems. Professor Deepadung notes that this College of Ayurvedic Medicine has the goal of preparing its graduates to practice the healing profession in a way which implements the strengths of both systems.

Dr. C.M. Francis provides a view of the Indian medical system that includes the philosophical and historical influences on which it is based. In a country which ranks as the second most populous and the largest democracy in the world, the socio-economic condition has a great influence on medical practices. Both ancient concepts and research developments from the West affect medical practice and ethics. As a result, the system is in flux.

The fundamental basis of medical ethics in India is the traditional concept of *ahimsa*, an ethical teaching which means a complete absence of ill-will to all beings. It comes from Hindu teachings which say that living beings are part of the divine Paratmatman, that it is only an illusion to believe that anyone is separated from anyone else. Since patient and doctor are part of the same unity, the conduct of the physician is to be motivated by agapic love.

Ayurveda is the ancient science of life and health which teaches the physician to approach the patient as a whole person and to engage in healing out of compassion. One who practices from this virtue-base can obtain the highest happiness because he or she has fulfilled his or her personal mission (*siddartha*). An ethics of trust between physician and patient is based on patient expectations of a value-system founded on such beliefs. Currently, however, an ethics of rights has been introduced and paternalistic approaches are being challenged. Mistakes in judgment are being questioned and informed consent procedures have been demanded. Philosophical acceptance of harms experienced (considering them to be one's karma) is gradually diminishing. The West has brought the increasingly accepted notion that people have the right to decide for themselves.

Among the conflicts which have arisen, as Professor Francis points out, is the problem of the purchasing of equipment from abroad which cannot be properly serviced. Physicians are trained at schools in the West and learn to use sophisticated diagnostic equipment which is ordered but not maintained. As in most other developing countries, the ethical problem then becomes: Ought developing countries to order such equipment which is unlikely to remain functioning and which must be bought with scarce foreign currency? Another difficulty, which places an ethical onus on suppliers, is the dumping of equipment, diagnostic test kits, and pharmaceuticals which are outdated or substandard and have been banned in other countries. Often these materials are sent to India even though they ought to be recalled and, in the case of pharmaceuticals, without even proper information concerning contraindications.

There is a great need for qualified health care personnel to provide services where they are unavailable. St. John's Medical College, Bangalore, and a few other medical colleges have addressed this problem by requiring that their medical graduates practice for a period of time in underserved areas.

The primary needs in India at present are the prevention and management of diseases of malnutrition and infection. The use of scarce foreign currency for sophisticated equipment, such as that used in centers for open heart surgery, is excluding a large part of the population from adequate basic health care. Other issues of medical ethics are related to the payment of poor women for surrogate motherhood and of poor persons for kidneys. Often non-Indians travel to India specifically for this purpose. About one hundred kidney transplants involving foreign patients are done every month.

Professor Francis notes that the changes in medical ethics involve moving away from precepts and practices of the ancients. Advances in science and technology and influences of other cultures have brought about a state of confusion when these issues are evaluated. He expresses the hope that there can be, with continuing effort, a judicious blending of the ancient and modern.

Zbigniew Bankowski characterizes the aim of physicians over the centuries as that of instituting a natural order and government in the parts of the body. This can be done best by integrating medical expertise with an understanding of the national, cultural, and religious context in which the patient lives.

A nation's health policy unerringly reveals the values that drive that society. Examination of the moral validity of such policies is of considerable importance not only to the society itself but also to the global community of which it is part. It is particularly important, however, to the individual who stands to benefit or suffer as a result of the policy and practices within his or her culture. Equitable distribution of medical resources and the just use of modern technology are primary considerations in any metaethical endeavor of this kind. As has been pointed out elsewhere, the three considerations which should motivate health policy and health policymakers are:

1. An attempt to control the social and economic impact of the unrestrained use of advanced medical technology in treating individual patients.
2. The achievement of a more equitable distribution of the benefits of medical knowledge, with just distribution varying according to many factors within the culture itself.
3. The use of medical knowledge in an anticipatory way for the collective good of present and future generations.

Since modern technology offers many possibilities, and each presents some conflict between social and individual good, medical policymakers face the important task of developing a strategy that optimizes the social uses of a nation's medical knowledge and resources. The notion of order which Dr. Bankowski proposed first in relation to the healing of the individual person, can be further applied at the global level. He introduced the notion of harmony, mentioned often during the conference, as the aim of dialogues of this kind whose purpose is to keep peace within divergent belief systems.

As Secretary General of the Council for International Organization of Medical Sciences (CIOMS), Dr. Bankowski began a series of international dialogues in 1985. The purpose of these meetings has been to provide a forum in which health policymakers may develop guides and justifications for choosing goals and priorities in the formation of health policy strategy. This series of dialogues gives policymakers the opportunity to formulate decisions which represent a resolution of diverse influences within their specific cultures as well as among differing cultures representing conflicting belief systems.

The diversity and richness of perspective in these contributions leaves us with a broad foundation for our emerging dialogue on global bioethics. It is more than just a work in comparative ethics. It is that. But it is also the beginning of the dynamic formation of a chain of reference in the global community.

Each contributor has been clear about the basic value of respect for life. And each has, in his own way, acknowledged the values of beneficence, autonomy, nonmaleficence, and justice.

One primary, recurrent pattern of concern has been the development of harmony as both component and evidence of health--within the body itself, in physician/patient/family relationships, and within the community in its wider and wider settings. The dialogue, then, is not to be seen as simply a forum for conflict resolution. It has greater potential. The real goal is that the continuing interchange of thought on bioethical issues may dynamically shape a flourishing global harmony in response to issues of common concern.

Patricia Mazzarella

2

Prologue: Intersections of Western Biomedical Ethics and World Culture

Edmund D. Pellegrino

Culture and ethics are inextricably bound to each other. Culture provides the moral presuppositions, and ethics the formal normative framework, for our moral choices. Every ethical system, therefore, is ultimately a synthesis of intuitive and rational assertions, the proportions of each varying from culture to culture. There is also in every culture an admixture of the ethnocentric and the universal, of that which is indissolubly bound to a particular geography, history, language, and ethic strain, and that which is common to all humans as humans.

These shaping forces, the intuitive and rational, the ethnocentric and the universal, are in constant flux within cultures. The specific point at which a balance is struck will vary from culture to culture. When cultures interact, these moral balance points are disturbed. A complex matrix of value intersections results. Where these balance points will be re-set in any particular culture is difficult to predict.

This is precisely the situation in contemporary biomedical ethics. In a world contracted in time and space by modern communications technologies, no people, however isolated or underdeveloped, can remain impervious to medical knowledge. Each culture is compelled to respond to both the potential advantages and the accompanying challenges to traditional values posed by humanity's new-found power over life, death, and procreation.

Whereas premature acceptance of these new technologies can threaten a culture's self-identity, premature rejection can deprive a culture of badly needed medical benefits. Each culture must decide how--and whether--to reconcile its own ethical system with what might be required to adapt to new medical technologies. This requires choosing what is congruent, and rejecting what is incongruent with deeply held beliefs about the nature, meaning, and purpose of human life.

In biomedical ethics, this transcultural challenge is vastly complicated because medical science and technology, as well as the ethics designed to deal with its impact, currently are Western in origin. They are deeply ingrained with three sets of values distinctly Western--the values of empirical science, principle-based ethics, and the democratic political philosophy. Such values are often alien, and even antipathetic, to many non-Western worldviews.

The dominant characteristics of Western science, ethics, and politics are mutually supportive: Western science is empirical and experimental, pursuing objectivity and quantification of experience. Ultimately, it attempts to control nature to the greatest extent possible. Western ethics is analytical, rationalistic, dialectical, and often secular in spirit. Western politics is liberal, democratic, individualistic, and law-governed. Western science, ethics, and politics provide an environment that gives rise to, and sustains, the use of complex medical technologies. As a result, it is difficult to divorce medical knowledge and the benefits it offers from the Western cultural and ethical milieu that supports and sustains it.

Western values, however, may be strongly at odds with worldviews held by billions of other human beings. Those billions may be less inclined to an aggressive uncovering of the mysteries of nature and less obsessed with the need for experimental verification. Instead, they may be drawn more strongly by the spiritual and qualitative dimensions of life. Their ethical systems may be less dialectical, logical, or linguistic in character, less analytical, more synthetic, or more sensitive to family or community consensus than to individual autonomy, more virtue-based than principle-based. In turn, their political systems may be more attuned to authority, tradition, ritual, and religion; more comfortable with, and more responsive to, the centralization of decision-making; more tolerant of social stratification and inequality.

Such divergences in value systems are often irreconcilable. Yet, as the power and influence of medical science and technology grow, these conflicting systems of belief will be drawn into more acute confrontation and conflict with each other. Only by dealing constructively with these conflicts can a nation enjoy the benefits of medical progress. Even more important, only in this way can we effect the transnational, transcultural cooperation necessary for the improvement of world health as a whole.

Such confrontations are evidenced in many technological, ethical, and cultural intersections. Some of these confrontations are more easily dismissed or neglected than others. In medicine, however, the issues are more urgent, less easily avoided, and more explicit than in other arenas. Moreover, disease has no respect for geographic or culture boundaries. As the biosphere expands to embrace the whole globe, every nation has a stake in every other nation's health. For these reasons, the practical and conceptual questions of transcultural biomedical ethics are more sharply defined than in some other domains of knowledge.

The central problem is the moral status of cultural autonomy. There would seem to be a *prima facie* obligation to respect cultural values that may differ from our own. Given even that *prima facie* obligation, we must, nevertheless ask ourselves: What are the limits of cultural autonomy? Is the limit reached only when one culture forcibly imposes its values upon another? Is cultural-ethical relativism the only valid moral posture? Are there morally valid and morally invalid cultures? Is there any foundation for a common morality by which different ethical systems may be judged and through which transcultural cooperative efforts can be transacted? Or, does it follow, as some would argue, that the quest for a common substantive ethics is futile in a pluralist world society? Are conceptual clarity and procedural guidelines all that ethics can be expected to provide? Does it then follow that medical and biomedical ethics are, themselves, purely cultural artifacts and that there should be as many medical ethical systems as there are cultures?

A strong case can be made for cultural autonomy and the obligation to respect ethical systems alien to our own. Culture is a complex whole which summates the most fundamental beliefs of a people in art, language, literature, custom, and law. It is gradually assimilated into every individual's personal identity from the moment that person begins to become aware of his or her cultural milieu. Even if we reject, or are rejected by, the culture in which we are born and raised, interaction with that culture will mold our deepest beliefs about the meaning and purpose of our political, communal, social, and individual lives. To violate a person's cultural beliefs and practices is tantamount to assaulting his or her very humanity. To impose alien beliefs and practices on an individual or an entire society is to violate their humanity. Such violations are immoral. Human beings, whether as individuals or aggregates, are inherently entitled to respect; they possess an inviolable dignity.

To grant this premise, however, is not to sanction the absolutization of either personal or cultural autonomy. While autonomy is to be respected, we must also recognize our interdependence--as individuals, cultures, societies, and states. The impact of medical technology cannot be contained within geographical or cultural boundaries. For that reason, absolutization of cultural autonomy is particularly dangerous in our use of medical knowledge. The impact of medical technology cannot be contained within geographical or cultural boundaries. Our capacity to prevent and cure illness, to forestall death, to be able to control procreation, to modify genes, to improve the lifespan, and ease disability has an enormous economic, political, and social impact on our world society.

Medical knowledge, like communication technology, makes the "global village" a reality. The central medical ethical issues we now face as individual countries are, or will shortly be, common problems. All countries want to take advantage of some feature of Western technology. Each will want to do so without compromising its own fundamental moral values. Yet what is accepted and what is rejected by one country has unavoidable effects on others. Cultural and ethical autonomy, therefore, must know some limit in the interest of world welfare.

The eradication of smallpox, for example, was not a Western but a world accomplishment. The science was Western. But if all nations had not cooperated in the massive vaccination of large populations all would have continued to be at risk, just as all are at risk, even today, whenever a contagious disease appears anywhere in the world. In the same way, responses to ethical issues in one part of the world are felt elsewhere: Effective but expensive life-saving treatments are not given equal moral weight. "Salvageable birth weight" varies enormously among countries, as do such practices as infanticide, sterilization, concern for the aged, infants, and children. Wealthy, organ-hungry countries can drain the organ supply of poorer countries by paying for organs. Wealthy nations can pursue clinical experimentation not permitted within their own borders by setting camp in countries with less rigorous surveillance. Confidentiality, patient autonomy, distributive justice are all interpreted differently in the professional mores of the world's physicians.

As we survey the spectrum of the world's moral perspectives depicted in this volume, we are struck simultaneously by the similarities and dissimilarities. The temptation is to concentrate on the extremes--emphasizing differences, which often foster claims to cultural superiority, or emphasizing similarities, which sacrifices moral integrity to ethical relativism. These extremes must be resisted. It is essential to seek the middle ground in which some values overlap. In this "middle ground" we must seek compromises which can be made without losing the whole of one's cultural identity.

There is reason to expect that such a shared moral ground may be found on some of the issues confronting contemporary biomedical ethics. We may take some solace in the historical fact that all major ancient cultures have had guidelines for the use of medical knowledge. Hippocratic, Chinese, Arabic, and Indian physicians shared an ethics based in the primacy of the patient's welfare. Each recognized that medical knowledge is not proprietary like other commodities, that those who possess it have moral obligations of a special kind, and that some suppression of self-interest in the interest of the sick person is a moral requirement of ethical practice.

These ancient premises have a continuing influence today. They find concrete expression in the ethical precepts of the Declarations of Helsinki and Geneva, the Ethical Codes of the World Medical Association, the International Code of Medical Ethics and the United Nations Principles of Medical Ethics, to name a few examples. Because they are shared across cultural systems, medicine and a concern for health are among the more accessible pathways for intercultural and transcultural discourse and cooperation. Physicians and other health care professionals can communicate in a common language across sociopolitical, historical, and cultural barriers that often isolate peoples from one another. That is the case because all health care professionals have experience of the ways in which medical knowledge may impinge on deeply ingrained cultural beliefs. They can also recognize ways in which traditional medical mores can be subverted by political and economic philosophy.

Despite the fact that, in many cultures, the physician's authority remains largely undisputed, patient autonomy, for example, is slowly becoming a reality. The growth and expansion of political democracy, education, and economic power are eroding the benign authoritarianism that was, for so long, the hallmark of professional medical ethics worldwide. In more cultures than ever before, there is recognition of the moral rights of patients to participate in decisions that affect them, to protection of confidentiality, to humane treatment, and access to health care. There is a long way to go before unanimity on these matters is achieved, but it is clear that older models of physician-dominated relationships are under scrutiny everywhere.

What emerges from the intersection of systems of medical ethics across cultural lines is a recognition of the need for, and the possibility of, some form of metacultural ethics which can ameliorate cultural relativism. In medical ethics, all ethical positions are not of equal moral status--regardless of how tightly bound they may be to a particular culture. Witness the approbation for cooperative efforts of physicians who oppose the use of nuclear weapons and the condemnation of physicians who torture or experiment with prisoners of war. Even if violations of patient rights are tolerated in certain social and cultural settings, they are not tolerable in any common ethics of medicine. Growing recognition of the moral rights of patients, their special vulnerability as sick persons, and the their dependency on the physician's knowledge constitute the empirical foundation of a morally defensible ethics of medicine. Those cultural systems that violate such norms cannot be given equal moral standing with systems which respect them. This is not because the cultural systems which support human and patients' rights are *per se* superior. Rather, it is because the protection of human rights is grounded in something more fundamental than culture--the deference owed to all human beings *qua* human beings. This is a norm by which every culture may be judged.

To be sure, the present idea of respect for the self-determination of patients originated in contemporary bioethics, which, in its present form, is a product of Western (largely American) conceptions of ethics. But, we must not forget that it has been only two decades since even Western medical ethics abandoned the stance of medical authoritarianism. It did so because it recognizes that the duty of respect for the moral right of patient autonomy is grounded in rights and moral claims all humans have on each other. It happens to have been first emphasized by "Western" medical ethics. But it should be recognized because of its metacultural justification, not its propagation by Western medicine. The dignity of the human person is not something that can be continually asserted or denied. It transcends culture because it resides inalienably in what it is to be a human being.

Indeed, the problem in the West is now becoming how to mitigate the absolutization of patient autonomy. Some bioethicists now argue that the physician is a mere instrument in the hands of the patient, that the physician's personal moral beliefs should be divorced from his professional life, and that the patient's wishes must be respected. This applies to such cases as active euthanasia, assisted suicide, abortion, purchase of organs for transplantation, all forms of reproductive technology and surrogate parenthood, preservation of confidentiality, or the use of public sources of health care funding. This form of absolute ethical individualism ignores the duties we owe others as members of the human community. Left unchecked, it would destroy any sense of communitarian ethics. And it would subvert the conscience of the physicians in morally dangerous ways.

Clearly, the Western--particularly the American--form of biomedical ethics must resist the forces within its own culture driving it to absolute individualism and moral atomism of a socially destructive kind. It must go beyond the tendencies within its own cultural milieu and seek something morally more fundamental. It must sift the conflicting values within democratic liberalism itself for those which have a morally valid foundation and those which do not. The physician must be recognized as a moral agent, as is the patient. The physician's moral beliefs cannot simply be set aside to satisfy the patient's demands. This question of balancing autonomy is today a necessary part of any transcultural dialogue in medical ethics.

The ethics of medicine offers a fruitful point for beginning a larger cultural dialogue between and among the world's major cultures. The ends of medicine are more easily defined than the ends of human life more generally. The functions of medicine derive from the needs of the sick person. These are easier to delineate than the more general needs of human beings as such for happiness or fulfillment. We cannot yet agree worldwide on a philosophical anthropology, but we probably can eventually agree on some philosophy of medicine and medical ethics suitable for resolving the dilemmas of medical progress if the dialogue is sustained and conducted with good will.

The ethical system of any culture is morally defensible because it is grounded in truths that transcend that culture; it is not morally defensible simply because it is the product of a particular culture. Respect for culture and ethics other than our own is the beginning of any intercultural dialogue, not its ending. The fact of cultural difference does not, as too many anthropologists have argued, necessitate absolute cultural relativism. Rather, it energizes the search for those ethical elements that transcend particular cultures.

Medical technology--and, parenthetically, political democracy--are reshaping the ancient edifice of medical ethics. As they come into closer contact with other world cultural and ethical systems they engender a dialectic and dialogue which is essential to the humane uses of medical knowledge. The wide variety of extant cultures and ethical systems notwithstanding, it seems clear that the emergence of a medical ethics based in certain features of our common humanity is possible and even likely.

As the transcultural dialogue in medical ethics continues, it should serve as an encouraging prototype for the larger dialogue between, and among, all cultural and ethical systems. This dialogue is needed if we are to find some metacultural set of moral values to which all may subscribe. This metacultural set of values means the triumph of some "superior culture." Its validity will be based in what it is to be a human being--over and above the particular language, art, custom, or history of any one people.

The papers in this volume highlight both the problems, and the potential for a dialogue among worldviews in medical ethics. The need to use medical knowledge humanely and within strict constraints can move us closer together or divide us further. Let us hope the dialogue continues and that medical ethics will serve to re-emphasize our shared fate as humans.

3

American Moralism and the Origin of Bioethics in the United States

Albert R. Jonsen

Since the early 1960s public and academic interest in ethical issues in medicine, the biosciences, and health care has flourished in the United States. This interest appeared here earlier than in other countries and has grown into a notable academic enterprise with extensive publications and conferences. It has become part of a wide range of public policy activities in which formal representation has been given to bioethical questions and bioethicists who assist in the development of legislation, regulations, and public policy. At least four major commissions have been established by Congress and many more committees have been appointed to deal with various ethical questions in biomedical science and practice.

One of the most recent of these public policy activities dealt with the problem of providing federal financial support to research involving the therapeutic use of human fetal tissue. In November, 1989, Dr. James Mason, Assistant Secretary for Health at the Department of Health and Human Services, rejected the recommendations of an ad hoc committee established to study the use of human fetal tissue for transplantation therapy of Parkinsonianism and diabetes. The committee had extensively studied the ethical aspects of the proposed procedure and, while recognizing certain serious problems, concluded that such a use could be considered ethically acceptable. Dr. Mason, to whom Secretary Sullivan had delegated final authority on this issue, rejected the committee's report. When he did so, he stated that his decision was "a matter of heart."[2]

Dr. Mason's words, undoubtedly sincere, reveal much about bioethics in the United States. In using the words "a matter of heart," he inadvertently recalled a moral tradition that runs wide and deep, although in our days rather silently, through American culture. I name that tradition, "American moralism." My thesis is that the tradition of American moralism at first fostered the concern about bioethics that appeared in the 1960s and grew with remarkable vigor in the next two decades. However, as nascent bioethics gradually was subsumed into the intellectual enterprise of academic ethics, the opinions of the bioethicists and the concerns of American moralism have grown increasingly divergent. My thesis is supported more by rough intuition than by refined research, but I believe that research would support that intuition. Anyone who would undertake the research would have to look more attentively at the history of the ideas I will sketch here, be more careful about the concepts I outline, and search out more thoroughly the texts that relate the events and ideas at the origins of bioethics in the decade between 1965-75, which I take as the formative decade of bioethics in the United States. This research, for the most part, remains to be done. In its absence, I will follow my intuition and set off on a rather bold, perhaps rash, exposition of my thesis about American moralism and bioethics.

I first propose what I take to be an uncontroversial premise: cultures have discernibly unique moralities, in the sense of explicit and implicit beliefs about the values that should inform personal and communal life. The designation, definition, and emphases on these values differ from culture to culture in varying degrees and at different times. I am confident in asserting this premise without further elaboration because I assume that this conference is based upon it. Each participant will, I imagine, describe bioethics in ways that match the moral beliefs of a specific culture, pointing out how certain ideas, say autonomy, are congenial to, or foreign to, a native morality. I will then go on to suggest that American moralism is American culture's matrix morality, that is, the deep source in which a certain way of thinking and feeling about the moral life is engendered and nourished.

The meaning I attribute to moralism is best explained by an historical and doctrinal excursus. In general, by moralism I mean a form of moral thought and expression characteristic of religious fundamentalism. However, by fundamentalism, I mean something more than the current phenomenon of popular evangelism, so enthusiastically embraced by many Americans and so criticized for its political involvement and for its own pitiful lapses into hypocrisy and exploitation. Contemporary fundamentalist religion is a pale imitation of a more powerful American religious tradition, one that had its roots in New England Puritanism and that dominated American culture throughout the nineteenth century. (The term "fundamentalism" is itself a twentieth century innovation).[1] But, alongside this native Protestant fundamentalism, an immigrant fundamentalism appeared and exerted its own powerful influence on American culture, namely, the moral theology of Irish Roman Catholicism marked by the doctrinal aberration called Jansenism. The Protestant and Catholic versions of moral fundamentalism have a common ancestry: the theology of John Calvin.

It is impossible in a short lecture to explicate fully the doctrinal and historical complexities of Calvinism, Puritanism, fundamentalism, and Jansenism. Permit me a rapid summary (which may, I fear, offend scholarly historians and theologians). In the seventeenth century, the Puritans, dissenters from Anglican ecclesiastical governance and influenced strongly by Calvinist theology, settled in New England. The history and the mentality of the Puritan settlers has been extensively described. Its foremost historian, Perry Miller, describes the Puritans' intent as "a society founded by men dedicated in unity and simplicity to realizing on earth eternal and immutable principles, and which progressively became involved with fishing, trade and settlement."[17] The clash between "eternal and immutable principles" and involvement with "fishing, trade and settlement" set a theme for American moralism that has persisted through this country's history.

The Puritan response was not to advise retreat from the world of secular activities, but to plunge into it with pure hearts. A clear, unambiguous perception of God's commandments and an unquestioning voluntary dedication to their observation would protect believers from contamination as they moved to subdue nature and society to the divine governance. This serene confidence found its intellectual counterpart in the moral philosophy taught at New England's first institution of higher learning, Harvard. The tenets of that moral philosophy were that "empirical and introspective study of human nature would lead to absolute standards and norms for human conduct . . . immutable divine law was as discoverable in ethics as in physics."[10] The moral philosopher Samuel Clarke profoundly influenced American moral philosophy, proclaiming that the believer could be led astray by "the created world (which) reveals inherent moral truths directly to man . . . this order is so logically fixed that God himself cannot but act and command in accord with it . . . only an imperfect and depraved understanding of the order, a will corrupted by particular interest or affection."[10]

Of course, depraved understanding and corrupt affections beset the human race, radically broken by sin. The will, or as was usually said, "the heart" must be continually purified. In the eighteenth century, the first Great Awakening, presided over by the religious genius Jonathan Edwards, summoned Americans to this purity of heart and dedication of life. Again, clear and unambiguous moral commandments were uttered; deep, affective response was demanded. It was less a matter of teaching people what they did not know than of reinforcing dedication to what was already known. In Edwards' words, "The informing of the understanding is all in vain any further than it affects the heart."[7]

Interrupted briefly by the Revolutionary War, the religious awakening revived in the first decades of the nineteenth century under the inspiration of Charles Finney. The revival meeting, at which manifest truths about salvation and morality were preached in vigorous and emotional terms and utter personal dedication was demanded, was the predominant method. As Miller wrote, "The dominant theme in America from 1800 to 1860 was the invincible presence of the revival technique . . . the revival . . . was a central mode of this culture's search for national identity . . . the task was to ascertain the sins of the community that needed reforming . . . to save the western migration from barbarism."[16]

Again, after the Civil War, revivalism in many new forms swept the country, presided over by Dwight Moody and Billy Sunday. The earlier fundamentalism, largely derived from Calvinist theology and Scottish common sense philosophy, preserved an intellectual heritage, in which reflection, guided by rightly ordered affection, revealed an immutable order of divine providence and moral truths. In this third period, fundamentalism ceded to the profoundly emotional, anti-intellectual religious sentimentalism that today goes by the name "fundamentalism." In this form, fundamentalism displays "an overwhelming emphasis on soul-saving, personal experience and individual prayer." To Dwight Moody, "most ideas seemed divisive and hence all but the least controversial were to be avoided."[14]

This quick, superficial history reveals a pattern. From the earliest settlement of North America to the present day, a powerful moral tradition has shaped the culture. That powerful tradition is Protestant fundamentalism, beginning as a Puritan application of Calvinist doctrine to the situation of the new world and developing as the insistent affirmation of clear, distinct moral principles, derived from the nature of things in which God's will was perceived and accepted by an affective, single-minded dedication of the heart. The most prominent evangelist of the Second Awakening, Charles Finney, affirmed that "everybody can agree upon the intellectual proposition. The only difference is that some grasp them with the heart and others with the mind. . . . holy angels and devils apprehend and embrace intellectually the same truths, yet how differently they are affected by them."[16]

However, America is more than the Protestant tradition flowing from the Puritans to the modern fundamentalists. Immigrant Catholicism provides its own moral culture. Strangely enough, it parallels the Calvinist tradition in spirit, if not in specifics. The first generation of American Catholics brought an English spiritual tradition to these shores, but rapidly, in the first decades of the nineteenth century, an immigrant clergy, many of them fleeing from the French Revolution, brought with them a spiritual and moral doctrine that was marked by Jansenism, a Catholic cousin of Calvinism. Calvin and Cornelius Jansen, a Belgian theologian, both found their spiritual inspiration in Augustine and both exploited the fideistic, voluntaristic, pessimistic notions of the greatest of the Western church fathers. The followers of Jansen denied Calvinist sympathies, but could not deny the similarity of concepts, logic, and inclinations that joined them to the Huguenots. "The type of piety that developed out of Jansenism," says the New Catholic Encyclopedia, "was inflexibly rigoristic . . . Jansenists were excessively moralistic and held that humanity had to be kept in check by penitential rigor."[11] A bitter theological and political battle raged over Jansenism in the French-speaking countries and in Rome and, even after Roman authorities formally condemned the doctrine at the close of the eighteenth century, it lingered deeply in the spirituality and theology of French Catholicism. Belgian missionaries brought it to the United States in the first decades of the nineteenth century.

Jansenism came in full force, however, with the waves of Irish immigrants from the 1820s until after the Civil War. Irish clergy, unable to be educated in British dominated Ireland, attended seminaries in France and Belgium (and to a lesser degree in Spain, which promoted its own brand of rigorism). The first seminary allowed to open in Ireland after the Ascendancy, St. Patrick's at Maynooth, was staffed by many professors educated at Louvain, where the university had always been sympathetic to Jansenism. In the very first year of its operation (1796), the faculty at Maynooth were warned by Roman authorities not to admit any liberal opinions in moral theology, repudiating "the excessive and wanton liberality of some in laying down the rules of morality, so that the mildness and suavity of evangelican charity shall never be disassociated from the salutary severity which is characteristic of Christian teaching."

The use of a text by a rigorist theologian was required. The liberal opinion that was to be repudiated was known as "probabilism," a doctrine despised by Jansenists and in fact permitted by the magisterium of the church. Maynooth sent a steady stream of missionaries to the Irish in America. John Tracy Ellis, dean of Catholic historians, writes: "If many of those of Irish birth or background in the United States continued . . . to display a strain of Jansenism in their thinking on moral issues such as problems connected with sex . . . it was no mystery where the ideas had taken their rise."[8] They had taken their rise in Irish seminaries staffed by clergy trained in Jansenist leaning institutions on the continent. They came, as well, from the thousands of nuns whose spiritual guidance and religious rules came from these clergy. Indeed, when American bishops sought to establish a seminary in Europe, to attract European clergy to serve in the United States, and to which promising young Americans could be sent for a European education, they selected Louvain (1857).

In the last half of the nineteenth century, American Catholicism embraced the techniques of revivalism that had long prevailed in Protestant fundamentalism. Groups of priests, specially trained in pulpit oratory, travelled from parish to parish, conducting "retreats" or "missions" at which powerful emotional appeals were made to convert sinners and revive religious fervor. A historian of the movement writes: "The stern moral code encouraged by the revival promoted an individual morality that blended with the evangelical thrust of the Catholic revivalism. Morality, not dogma, right doing, not correct believing, was the thrust of the revival method . . . preachers impressed upon people what must be done, or more often, what must be avoided in order to gain salvation . . . revivalists sought a change of heart, not a change of opinion."[6] Thus, at the same time in American life, Protestants and Catholics, who otherwise wished nothing more than to be distinct from each other, were engaged in a similar program: the encouragement of moralism, rigid in content and emotive in tone.

The similarities between Protestant fundamentalism and Irish Jansenism are many. For our purposes, the most important are the insistence on clear, unambiguous moral principles, known to all persons of good faith. Both deny the possibility of moral paradox or irreconcilable conflict of principles. Fundamentalism cannot accept the possibility of Kierkegaardian moral conflict, for the righteous God cannot command (as He seems to have commanded Abraham) to obey and, at the same time, to do a moral evil. Conflict must be explained as only apparent, never as real paradox.[21]

Both fundamentalisms avoid, as much as possible, detailed examination of exceptions to principles and rules. Exceptions to principle may come from an occasional "miraculous" suspension of divine command, but more likely are a symptom of sinful weakness of will. Probabilism, the doctrine that a moral problem can be understood in diverse ways and that differential moral judgments can be offered, is repudiated. Casuistry, the technique of moral analysis of particular cases, is despised in Calvinism and converted into legalism in Jansenist Catholicism.[12] Both have a strong tendency to lump complex moral problems into simple, overarching ideas and to link together issues which, viewed from a more discerning viewpoint, appear distinct. For example, contraception and abortion are inextricably linked in Jansenist thinking; sex education and pornography are equated in Protestant fundamentalism.

It might be suspected that "the slippery slope," one of the favorite ethical arguments in current usage, derives from, or is at least congenial to, American moralism. This argument, closely inspected, seems to assert that while the actual case or issue at hand might be morally acceptable, analogous cases would not be, and thus, the actual case must be prohibited. The move from the actual to the analogous comes, not through logical or conceptual connections, but from the weakness of will of persons, who are very unlikely to resist the temptation to perform the unacceptable, once the acceptable is allowed them. This distrust of human moral strength is profoundly Jansenistic and Calvinistic.

I have spoken primarily about the moral forms of Calvinism and Jansenism: they both proclaimed that moral truths were clear, discernable to all of pure heart; they both affirmed absolute moral principles, from which any departure must be counted as sinful, making little or no room for justifiable exception. The actual content of those principles varied, but both traditions heralded the ten commandments as dominant, both cherished strictly ordered plans of life, both were overconcerned with sexuality, both attacked intemperance by proposing, not temperance, but abstinence, both promoted to absolutist moral status certain virtues, such as patriotism, while ignoring others, such as tolerance.

In the long history of these traditions, the moral inflexibility sometimes achieved moral victories of great note. Abolitionism, untempered by concern for social and economic consequences, was a Calvinist moral victory. Other battles urged by moral absolutism, such as Prohibition, were miserable moral defeats. Moralism is absolutist in the etymological sense, namely, in abstraction from any actual circumstances. The principles are correct in themselves and must be affirmed: exceptions and excuses must not be considered extensively because such considerations would distract from the principle itself. Indeed, as Calvin himself once noted, casuistry is to be condemned because its consideration of a variety of exceptions and excuses "deepens anxiety."[5]

In fact, the theological father of both fundamentalisms displayed an attitude that prevails even in his most remote progeny. One of his sympathetic biographers has described that attitude: "He tended to feel uneasy if he could not organize his understanding of the world by dividing phenomena neatly into antithetical categories: black and white, darkness and light, we and they, insiders and outsiders. . . . he relieved his fear of the abyss by cultural constructions, boundary systems and patterns of control that might help him recover his sense of direction. . . . his moralism found expression in his characteristic vocabulary of order and disorder, purity and contamination."[4]

American moralism also sees the world in antithetical categories and seeks boundary systems and patterns of control that will affirm order against disorder. This is a moralism that fits the experience of a people settling a new land, moving into the western wilderness, immigrating to a strange country among religious and ethnic strangers, affirming individual liberty and social cohesion at the same time. Out of a strange and dangerous land, they forged a familiar, orderly place. The farm replaced the forest and law and order dominated violent chaos.

I am proposing that the confluence of these two streams, flowing from the same source in Calvinist-Augustinian thought, has watered the ground of American culture. The crop that they produce is a strain of moral thinking that deeply believes in clear, unambiguous moral principles, in the ability of common sense to grasp those principles (when common sense is not clouded by self-interest), in the importance of the observance of these principles for the common good of the community. However, the stream beds through which coursed these great rivers of thought are now quite dry: they are, in effect, like the deep canyons of the Southwest, traces of waterways that indelibly mark the landscape.

This metaphor suggests that contemporary American culture is unaware of the sources of its moralism, although the marks made by those sources are manifest. In modern America, moral behaviors seem to represent wide pluralism; the rigidity of the Calvinist and Jansenist heritage seems dissolved into vague tolerance for all but the most outrageous violations. Indeed, an argument can be made that American moralism has been so thoroughly repudiated that nothing remains of it but ridicule. Still, I believe that the moralism generated by those traditions survives in the form, if not the content of the American mentality. The recent upsurge of interest in ethics in all aspects of American life flows, I think, in the river beds cut by the old traditions.

We are dealing today with the secular remnant of this deep fundamentalism: we may speak of a "secular fundamentalism." This describes the same absolutism, the same dichotomous world of good and bad, right and wrong, but shorn of its religious rationale and of its religious sanctions. Contemporary Americans may consider themselves morally liberal, broad-minded, even uncommitted, yet when pressed on a moral question, strains of the old moralism will appear. The fundamentalism of Calvin, the Awakenings and Jansenism had as its rationale what Calvin himself called "the first use of the law," namely, to convict men of their failure to live up to the righteousness of God. It is, he wrote, "a mirror ... in which we see our iniquity" and are driven to repentance.[5] Such a use of the law demands absolute adherence; it can brook no exceptions or excuses. Secular fundamentalism is equally as rigid but without the religious rationale: it is rigidity that has lost its meaning. Religious fundamentalism was also sanctioned by God's reward and punishment. One could win heaven or deserve hell; no middle place was available (Jansenists could stop over in purgatory, but only for peccadillos, of which there were not many). Secular fundamentalism retains the ominous seriousness of obedience to the law, but lacks the sanctions of eternal reward and punishment. It is, then, a secular morality, a secular fundamentalism: law, rule, and principle detached from religious rationale and sanction.

What has this to do with bioethics in the United States? I maintain that the original interest in bioethical issues grew out of American moralism. I do not mean that contemporary fundamentalism had anything to do with the emergence of bioethics: it essentially ignored these issues with the exception of abortion and contraception. I do mean that the remnants of American moralism as they form the characteristic way Americans think about morality had a great deal to do with the origins of bioethics.

The innovative and the unfamiliar stimulate the response of American moralism: how is this new thing or thought to be drawn into the ordered and clear structure of moral principles? If the world reveals moral truth to the conscientious (the secular substitute for devout) observer, what does this new thing in the world tell us of moral order? Where is it to be subsumed under the plan of clear and unambiguous principles? Obviously, the ambiguity of the new is intolerable and must be reduced to the clarity of the familiar and accepted.

The actual history of the emergence of bioethics in the United States remains to be written. In the absence of that record, we can start the history where we choose. The options are multiple: the selection of patients for chronic hemodialysis in Seattle in 1962, Beecher's accusation of unethical research in 1966, the initiation of heart transplants in 1969, or the revelation of the Tuskeegee and Willowbrook experiments in 1972. Clearly, the interest was strong enough to support the foundation of the Hastings Center in 1969 and the Kennedy Institute in 1970.

Certainly, one crucial event was the publication of Paul Ramsey's book *Patient as Person* in 1970.[22] That book gave a context, arcane and turgid, but passionate and reasoned, to the emerging concerns. Properly, the book was written by a man steeped in the theology of Calvin and Edwards and revealed a mind as anxious as Calvin's to bring order to the new chaotic features of contemporary medical science. Ramsey was more comfortable with the title "moralist" than the newfangled "ethicist." His concerns were clearly within the stream of American moralism: he sought principles to bring clarity into confusion and, while admitting room for exceptions, made that room as narrow as possible. The Biblical concept of covenant was as important to him as a theme of moral order as it was to his Puritan ancestors.

A second event of importance was personal: I was asked to serve on the Totally Artificial Heart Assessment Panel, formed by Dr. Theodore Cooper, Director of the National Heart and Lung Institute in 1972. This was the first formal acknowledgment of the nascent bioethics movement by the federal government. The panel was asked to assess the "ethical and moral implications of the totally implantable artificial heart," then under study at the institute and in several research institutions. I have described the process of this panel and my own contribution to it elsewhere.[13] For our purposes here, however, only one point is relevant: the search for "ethical and moral implications" of this and of other new technologies was likely to diverge from American moralism. Questions were latent in the problem of the artificial heart that required something more than application of principles. The totally implantable heart was powered by an implanted nuclear power device. It was not easy, for example, to find a moral formula that would help in balancing the benefits of several years of continued life for the recipient of the heart against the risks of radiation-induced cancer to other unassociated persons.

The Artificial Heart Assessment Panel was followed by a second, major investment of the federal government in bioethics. Congress established the National Commission for the Protection of Human Subjects of Biomedical and Behavioral Research. In the wake of several alleged abuses of subjects by researchers, Congress directed the commission to devise ways to protect the rights and welfare of subjects of research. Among the Congressional mandates was the instruction to study the "principles governing biomedical research." The commission responded to that instruction by producing the Belmont Report in which the ethical principles of beneficence, respect for autonomy, and justice were applied to the activities of research.

As a commissioner, I participated in the formulation of that report (in fact, its first draft was formulated at a small gathering of commissioners and consultants in my study in San Francisco). Today, I am dubious of its status as a serious ethical analysis. I suspect that it is, in effect, a product of American moralism, prompted by the desire of Congressmen and of the public to see the chaotic world of biomedical research reduced to order by clear and unambiguous principles. However, the commission realized that, despite the statement of principle, the problems posed by doing research in an ethical manner went beyond principle. They were essentially casuistic: requiring a method and mechanism for inspecting each problem on its own terms. Thus, the commission endorsed the Institutional Review Board as the casuistic forum in which principles would be tested against special circumstances. The IRB is by far more important ethically than the Belmont Report.[18, 19]

A similar reflection could be made on the President's Commission for the Study of Ethical Problems in Medicine, on which I also served. Among the many problems studied by that commission, one must suffice to illustrate my thesis. The commission was satisfied that sound ethical analysis demonstrated that no moral obligation could be imposed to provide life support for persons in the clinical condition called "persistent vegetative state."[20] We believed that this conclusion would be readily accepted by professionals, by the public, and by the law. Indeed, it was among the first few cases to come to public attention. However, in the last several years, the matter has become controversial, primarily over the question of the withdrawal of nutrition and hydration. The decision of the Supreme Court of the United States in the matter of Nancy Cruzan on 25 June 1990 is a precedent-setting moment in the development of thought on this matter. Yet, the ethical reasoning developed to justify the original proposition remains unchallenged in concept and in logic. Ethical argument has encountered American moralism.

The first manifest resurgence of the moralistic mentality occurred when the Ethical Advisory Board of the National Institutes of Health submitted its report on in vitro fertilization.[9] Having been requested by the secretary of DHEW to advise on the ethics of providing federal research funds for in vitro fertilization, the newly established body, made up of physicians, scientists, ethicists, and others did a careful review of the arguments pro and con. They concluded that in vitro fertilization studies should be supported. Their report was ignored by all authorities in the departmental hierarchy; no funding has ever been provided to this day. It can be opined that one point, namely, the problem of disposition of fertilized but unimplanted embryos, stymied the official response. To tolerate discard of these embryos would be, in the minds of a fundamentalist, tantamount to abortion; abortion is forbidden; therefore, in vitro fertilization is forbidden. This is the response of American moralism to the nuanced casuistry of the ethicist consultants.

The incident with which this essay opened, namely, Dr. Mason's rejection of the deliberations of the ad hoc committee on fetal tissue transplantation now comes into focus. Dr. Mason responded to a message from his "heart." I'm sure he did not appreciate the Augustinian, Calvinist, Edwardian, and Jansenist overtones of his expression. Still, his decision echoed American moralism. There are clear and unambiguous principles touching all aspects of life. They are known not by the intellect but by the heart. As such, they are profoundly personal, although, strangely, open to all conscientious persons in the moral community. This is American moralism. The committee's report, on the other hand, was a product of ethics, an intellectualist, casuistic exercise that dissolved the clarity of principle and exalted exceptions and consequences over unbreachable rule and immutable value. Thus, Dr. Mason was listening in his conscience to the advice of Jonathan Edwards, "the informing of the understanding is all vain any further than it affects the heart."

I am suggesting that the original impetus for bioethics came from an American moralism that sought to bring the chaos of the new scientific medicine into the order of moral principle. However, the task of doing this fell into the hands of persons who had studied philosophy and theology in quite a different tradition than Calvinist fundamentalism and Jansenist Catholicism. The small group of scholars in the first generation of bioethicists were skeptics within the culture of moralism. They were the intellectuals whom the old fundamentalists so mistrusted. The moral philosophers and moral theologians who became the first bioethicists had read logical positivists, pragmatists, utilitarians, and existentialists. Protestant theologians among them were disciples of the Niebuhrs and readers of Kierkegaard. Catholic theologians were struggling free of the legalism and authoritarianism that had entrapped Catholic moral theology. Clarity of method was more salient an issue than clarity of principle; moral ambiguity was more respectable a stance than moral certitude (Fr. Richard McCormick's first major contribution was a small book entitled *Ambiguity in Moral Choice*).[15] While in the beginning, the misfit was not noted, it has become slowly manifest. Today, ethical analysis done by the moral philosophers and theologians who do bioethics is much more likely to produce "probabilistic" opinions, that is, a range of options that enjoy greater or less probability in terms of the strength of rational argument and logic that support them. This is dismaying to American moralism. The recent collapse of the attempt to establish a Congressional Bioethics Commission and the failure to have re-established the Ethics Advisory Board may be symptoms of the misfit. The work of ethicists can no longer be expected to uphold the clear and unambiguous principles of American moralism. Those who affirm these principles can only suffer from Calvinist anxiety in the presence of those more likely to allow exceptions than to uphold principles.

There is a peculiar expression abroad in American discourse about ethics: almost inevitably, the phrase "moral and ethical" appears. I have never known quite what to make of the linking of these two words. They are, viewed etymologically, synonyms, meaning respectively in Latin and in Greek, the same, namely, custom. Scholars suggest distinctions, such as that moral refers to actual behavior and beliefs and ethics to the academic discipline that studies morality. Still, the linkage of the two is somewhat puzzling. Now, although I cannot explain it, I can glimpse some use for it.

Let us suggest that they are linked because there are really two tasks to be accomplished in dealing with any moral problem in the United States. One of them is to describe as fully and accurately as possible the moral dimension, that is, the way the problem appears within the preview of American moralism. This is primarily a sociological task, in the fashion of Bellah's *Habits of the Heart*.[3] The second is to apply to the problem the intellectual techniques of analysis known as ethics. In the twenty years of bioethics, the second task has been done rather well; the former has been done fitfully and poorly. For many problems, the split has not led to any serious disagreement: the moral view of personal self-determination and the philosophical concept of personal autonomy blend rather nicely in the doctrine of informed consent. In other problems, such as the ones mentioned above, the split has led to apparently irreconcilable differences. We attribute these too casually to "political differences." They are, rather, the pervasive effect of American moralism which is, at certain points, unshakably resistant to the intellectual analysis done by some of Jonathan Edward's devils, who may be, in this case, the bioethicists.

NOTES

1   Averill L.J. *Religious Right. Religious Wrong.* New York: Pilgrim Press, 1988.
2   Ban extended on research using fetal tissue. *Seattle Post Intelligencer*, Nov. 2, 1989, 1.
3   Bellah R. *Habits of the Heart*. Berkeley: University of California Press, 1985.
4   Bouwsma J.W. *John Calvin. A Sixteenth Century Portrait.* Oxford: Oxford University Press, 1988.
5   Calvin J. *Institutes of the Christian Religion*, vol. III, Philadelphia: Westminster Press, 1960.
6   Dolan J. *Catholic Revivalism. The American Experience 1830-1900*. Notre Dame: University of Notre Dame Press, 1978.
7   Edwards J. A Treatise on religious affections. In: Smith J., ed. *Works of Jonathan Edwards*, vol 2. New Haven: Yale University Press, 1959.
8   Ellis J.T. The formation of the American priest: a historical perspective. In: Ellis J.T., ed., *The Catholic Priest in the United States*. Collegeville, MN: St.John's University Press, 1971.
9   Ethics Advisory Board, Department of Health, Education, and Welfare. *Support of Research Involving Human in vitro Fertilization and Embryo Transfer.* Washington DC:US Government Printing Office, 1979.
10   Fiering N. *Moral Philosophy at 17th Century Harvard*. Williamsburg: University of North Carolina Press, 1981.
11   Jansenism, *The New Catholic Encyclopaedia*, vol. 7, New York: McGraw-Hill, 1967; 825.
12   Jonsen A.R., Toulmin S.E. *The Abuse of Casuistry.* Berkeley: University of California Press, 1988.
13   Jonsen A.R. The totally implantable artificial heart. *Hastings Center Report* 1973, 3: 1-3.
14   Marsden G.M. *Fundamentalism in American Culture*. New York: Oxford University Press, 1980.
15   McCormick R. *Ambiguity in Moral Choice*. Milwaukee: Marquette University Theology Department, 1973.
16   Miller P. *The Life of the Mind in America*. New York: Harcourt, Brace, 1965.
17   Miller P. *The New England Mind*. Cambridge: Harvard University Press, 1962.
18   National Commission for the Protection of Human Subjects of Biomedical and Behavioral Research. *The Belmont Report.*, Washington DC: U.S.Government Printing Office, 1978.
19   National Commission for the Protection of Human Subjects of Biomedical and Behavioral Research. *Institutional Review Boards*. Washington, DC: U.S. Government Printing Office, 1978.
20   President's Commission for the Study of Ethical Problems in Medicine and in Biomedical and Behavioral Research. *Deciding to Forego Life Sustaining Treatment*, Washington DC: U.S.Government Printing Office, 1983.

21 Quinn P. Moral obligation, religious demand and practical conflict. In: Aude R., Wainwright W.J., eds. *Rationality. Religious Belief and Moral Commitment*. Ithaca: Cornell University Press, 1986.

22 Ramsey P. *The Patient as Person*. New Haven: Yale University Press, 1970.

4

Minority Perspectives on Biomedical Ethics

Robert F. Murray, Jr.

INTRODUCTION

I should make it clear at the outset that I consider myself to be a student of applied ethics more than anything else. Most of the ideas and insights I will propose in this paper have been gathered during the course of two conferences which explored the topic: Black Perspectives in Bioethics. The first was held in February of 1987 and the second in December of 1989. It has been rather a small step to extend my thinking from the foundation of insights developed by the scholars who presented their ideas at those meetings to include similar ideas and concepts relevant to other minority groups. (By other minority groups I refer to ethnic groups of color, e.g., Hispanic, Asian, and Native American groups). What I present here probably ought to be considered a commentary on "work in progress" since the long range plan of the co-conveners of that series of meetings, Drs. Harley Flack and Edmund Pellegrino, is that a body of moral and ethical analysis be developed and promulgated based on clearly articulated ethical and moral principles that arise out of the ethnic and cultural traditions of peoples of African origin. This is no mean task and will occupy the scholars who have committed themselves to this goal for some years to come. In the meantime I'd like to share just a few of the embryonic ideas that are being developed by myself and many others. In keeping with the goals of the conference I will consider the ethical values that are pre-eminent in the African-American community and how such values are ranked; I will also consider the basis for differences in the approach to and the resolution of particular biomedical dilemmas.

BACKGROUND

It is generally acknowledged that human behavior is always influenced more or less by the culture in which it operates. Not only human behavior but also basic moral and ethical values are subject to cultural influence (Kluckhohn and Strodtbeck, 1973). In a large and heterogeneous society like the United States, subgroups or minorities follow behavior patterns that differ from that of the majority group. Their orientations appear to be conditioned by their culture, which will often, in specific instances, vary considerably from group to group.

These orientations are also subject to the influence of the basic ethical and moral values of the group. There may also be some variation in value orientation within minority groups since there may be subcultural differences within ethnic groups. Of course the degree of such variation will be a function of how broadly the ethnic or cultural group is defined. Knowing the degree of such ethnic variation within group diversity is important if one wishes to define cultural norms for a specific ethnic or cultural group. In the course of the initial workshop, a diverse group of African-American scholars and health care professionals reached a consensus that there was an African-American perspective in biomedical ethics which required further exploration.

Further, it was felt that this was derived from the unique nature of the African-American experience which has been shaped by the experience of "slavery, segregation, discrimination, poverty and a disadvantaged position with respect to education, health and medical care." This formulation grew out of the consideration of a concept known as "moral pluralism," the designation of the idea that the views held by a group of people, however defined, of what is good and bad, right and wrong, may legitimately differ from those held by other groups and further, that the differences often derive from a variation in the cultural values, customs, norms, and the "world view" of the groups whose morals are being compared. Since minority groups, in general, and African-Americans, in particular, emerged from an historical and contemporary experience which differed significantly from that of other ethnic groups, and especially the dominant Euro-American group in the United States, a moral philosophy has been developed that is unique to them. It appeared that a particular set of issues and questions should be explored that would further define the foundations of the African-American ethical and moral framework. These issues include the following:

1.   What are the pre-eminent ethical and moral principles that influence the culture?
2.   What is the concept of personhood in a particular culture?
3.   How is "health" or the state of "wellness" defined?
4.   What is the culturally derived relationship between the patient and the healer? How do they interact?

If reliable and valid answers to these questions are found, it is highly likely that the basis for many of the problems that now confront and confound those who operate the health care system can be understood and possibly be partially or fully resolved. Programs which are supposed to attack health care problems in a particular ethnic group can be designed and implemented in a manner that is consistent with the value systems of the group that is to be served by them.

Ethical Values in African-Americans

At the most recent conference convened to explore the foundations of the African-American perspective in bioethics (December 1989), a consideration of the theological basis for the difference between African-American and Euro-American religious values was presented by Professor Cheryl Saunders of the Howard University School of Religion. She considered the question of whether, if there is a black bioethic there isn't also a "black theology." The concept of black or African-American theology is similar to and closely tied to "liberation theology" which focuses on the freeing of the human spirit. Such a theology begins with an analysis and understanding of oppression, then affirms the personhood of the oppressed persons and finally shows the direction to be taken for liberation. The concept may not be limited to the experience of any one group but fits closely with the experience that African-Americans have had with slavery and then racism. She proposes that it is this "black" or "liberation" theology which has strongly influenced the development of ethical and moral principles affecting African-Americans today. A reason for this is that, historically, the church has had a central role in the development and shaping of the ethical values in the black community. Following from this, Professor Saunders lays out contrasting cultural differences between Euro- and African-Americans that helps one to understand certain of the ethical differences. It is obvious that these concepts are highly relative when they are applied to a group. They are meant to indicate strong tendencies or predominant themes in the literature or art or behavioral norms of large segments of the group. Contrasting differences of this sort can also be recognized in other ethnic groups.

African-American Ethos	Euro-American Ethos
Holistic	Particularistic
Inclusive	Exclusive
Communalistic	Individualistic
Strongly spiritual	Intellectual (secular)
Strongly theistic	Agnostic or atheistic
Improvisational approach	Structured approach
Humanistic	Materialistic

If these relative value differences can be accepted for the sake of discussion, differences in the ranking of ethical values that have been proposed by the African-American working group can be more readily understood.

There is general agreement that there is one set of ethical principles affecting all aspects of health care for everyone. These are autonomy, justice, beneficence, and nonmaleficence. Viewed against the backdrop of their history in this country, and as a result of the oppression and dehumanization experienced during slavery, and the Reconstruction, the effects of these experiences are still influencing the behavior and values of African-Americans today. In the opinions of the participants in the 1987 conference on African-American bioethical perspectives, the ethical principle of *justice* will be most highly valued by this group of people, whereas *autonomy* is given much greater weight in the Euro-American and other cultures. This assessment is not based on a scientific survey and it is possible that a survey taken of a representative sample of African-Americans would show that most would rank one of the other values more highly. There are other ethical values that may be considered in conjunction with these principles which include security, survival, and general welfare.

There have been two other reported attempts to identify the ethical perspectives of some minority groups, including African-Americans, concerning population policy in the first case and human experimentation in the second case.

The first study was carried out as a project of the Research Group on Ethics and Population of the Institute of Society, Ethics, and the Life Sciences (now known as the Hastings Center) at the request of the National Commission on Population Growth and the American Future which had been established in March 1970 (Veatch, 1977). Analyses of the perspectives on ethics and population policy of black Americans, Spanish-surname Americans, Native American Indians, and women were considered. This research group spent three years (1970-1973) performing these studies. As a member of that task force I performed the analysis of black Americans and found at that time, in a survey of the literature and conversations with representatives of groups with predominantly black support, that the current dominant value was self-determinism. The Black Power Movement had achieved considerable momentum and the considerable gains of the civil rights movement were still being enjoyed during this period. Although full equality hadn't been achieved, African-Americans had been tasting the fruits of justice and had reason to believe that the progress they had realized toward full citizenship would be permanent. The values listed in order of their perceived relative importance to black Americans at that time was:

- Security/survival
- Power/self-determination
- Truth-telling
- Justice

Central to proposed population policy were aggressive programs of birth control. These programs were seen as genocidal by many black groups and as threatening by Hispanic and Native American minorities as well. It is for this reason that security/survival and self-determination may have been placed at the top of the list of values. These concerns were not without justification in the views of many leaders in the black community at that time. It should be noted that autonomy as such was not listed.

Another important concept which became apparent in the course of this study was the considerable degree of heterogeneity in the black community. At least eight political and religious groups were identified whose opinions had to be taken into account. One of the small but highly vocal groups (which no longer exists) is the Black Panther Party. As is the case in any defined group of this sort, the heterogeneity of these groups complicates attempts to determine which values they favor.

The second major effort to identify ethical perspectives in minorities took place as part of the studies carried out under the auspices of the National Commission for the Protection of Human Subjects of Biomedical and Behavioral Research. The commission sponsored a National Minority Conference on Human Experimentation to identify minority perspectives on the ethics of human experimentation which was held in January of 1976 in Reston, Virginia. Speakers at the conference discussed the infamous Tuskegee experiments, psychosurgery, psychological testing of minorities, the use of drugs in behavior modification,and various aspects of health care delivery. The major ethical emphases in the conference were on informed consent, privacy and confidentiality, and the delivery of health care. But, running throughout the presentations at the conference was the theme of self-determination. Many members of the conference reported instances in which African-Americans and other minorities experienced dehumanizing experiences in experimental settings and in health care. These experiences prompted them to require that members of the minority communities involved in programs of experimentation and of health care delivery be involved in decisionmaking capacities and in the review of such programs in order to safeguard these individuals from abuse and dehumanization.

As a result of this conference and subsequent deliberations the National Commission, in a report "Ethical Guidelines for the Delivery for Health Services by DHEW," made specific recommendations to assure privacy of individuals receiving health services under programs conducted or supported by DHEW (previously DHHS). The commission also recommended that the rights and responsibilities of patients receiving health services be explained to them in language appropriate to their backgrounds; that professional committees monitor practices in all health service facilities supported by DHEW; and that programs be supported which promote both the training of increased numbers of minority individuals to serve at all levels in the health professions and the education of health professionals in ethical and social issues (1978).

It is of interest that a symposium to discuss the ethical implications of human experimentation was held under the sponsorship of the National Academy of Sciences in 1976. The Tuskegee experiment is not mentioned at all in the report of that conference. This may be an indication of the insensitivity to the minority perspective on bioethics which existed at that time.

Because of the long history of suffering, dehumanization, and deprivation there is among African-Americans an emphasis on the desire to satisfy needs immediately and to seek rapid relief of suffering. The focus on living *carpe diem* and not postponing gratification is a way for people in distress to maintain hope, especially when they live under conditions from which there seems to be no escape. They don't set long-term goals and don't adopt an ethical stance that leads to delayed gratification. There is also an intellectual allegiance to black African roots that emphasizes allegiance to the group and a sharing of resources. The concept of "self" is equated with that of "community." This is influenced to some degree by the values of the dominant society. There is an emotional commitment to a capitalistic ethic. The existence of an affluent African-American elite presents a dilemma which conflicts with the notion that justice is most highly valued. Furthermore, the typical symbols of law and order may not be respected because they often serve as the source of repression rather than protection of life and limb.

In this context, African-Americans value the "good life" as one in which they are able to enjoy a rich and fulfilling spiritual and emotional life in close relationships to friends and family, with a minimum of intellectual restraints. Even the traditional African-American church is a place to "have a good time" as indicated by the joy often expressed in the spirituals and gospel music so frequently performed. This contrasts with the generally "serious" tone of services in the Euro-American churches. A certain amount of this same spirituality and emotionality can be seen in the Hispanic and Native American cultures.

ETHICAL ISSUES IN HEALTH AND HEALTH CARE

All the studies of health statistics in African-Americans and other minorities indicate clearly that these peoples, with only a few exceptions, lag far behind the white majority in the quality of their health (Heckler, 1985; CDC Report, 1989). Not only are the health parameters of blacks inferior, but in some types of illness, e.g., cancer and stroke, they are getting worse. In the view of many analysts, this discrepancy is primarily due to a lack of adequate access to health care for African-Americans. Since there is a strong emphasis on immediate response and relief of pain, African-Americans are unlikely to focus on or be interested in wellness and prevention, especially those in the lower socioeconomic groups. This is part of the different and distinctive worldview that is reflected in the literature and the music of black Americans.

Generally, people will be able to get health care if they are able to pay for it. Unfortunately, those in greatest need of health care are those least likely to get it. Those who are poor and are dependent on government funding are likely to get the least effective care. Those who pay will tend to determine the quality of health care that is delivered. The most recent examples are the HMOs and their determination of the rules under which bills are paid. Those who are best able to pay the required health insurance premiums will get the best and most prompt service.

Health care providers have to respond to the perceived needs of African-American patients even when there are significantly different moral foundations between patients and health professionals. Black patients want most of all to be treated fairly and to be accorded the highest possible quality of care. When there are serious or significant moral disputes between patients and health caregivers, such disputes can be resolved by an appeal to the hospital ethics committee. This committee must have, as members, persons who are representatives of the non-medical community.

In order to realize the fruits of a fair application of the principle of justice in the health care setting one can appeal to the basic provisions of the United States Constitution, which guarantees the rights of all its citizens. But the African-American and other minority communities should be instructed concerning their rights, and, furthermore, they need to know how to secure those rights. The Constitution, which was written to exclude black Americans from its provisions is, all too often, still interpreted in ways that minimize their access to certain of its major provisions. In the final analysis, unless there is a significant reform in the system of justice in the United States, this document will not be the vehicle through which minority peoples achieve both their full status as citizens and reliable access to health care.

In the most recent of the symposia designed to explore major ethical perspectives in the light of the African-American experience and the African tradition, there was a significant beginning to much needed study and analysis of the degree to which their African roots have influenced the contemporary value systems of African-Americans and other minority groups. There is a special need to develop a long-term program to continue these studies and to publish and disseminate their results so that they will be available to people who are making health care policy decisions. The ethical conflicts that exist or threaten to develop must be studied and remedial actions must be considered so that the intercultural tensions that exist can be reduced. Positive relations should be forged between the African-American majority and the powers that be. As the historical and socioeconomic status of the parameters of the bioethical perspective of black Americans is further developed, the connections to their African roots will become more distinct.

The longer the question is studied, the more convincing the evidence for an African-American perspective in biomedical ethics becomes. But a certain amount of caution should be exercised lest the distinctions that are identified between African-Americans and Euro-Americans become ammunition for the use of people who wish to promote racist ideals and thinking and so further isolate, oppress, and dehumanize African Americans. Tremendous progress has been made toward achieving the status of full citizenship for black Americans since World War II. Some of the progress made has been eroded during the last eight years by an unsympathetic administration. It is critical that minority groups continue working to regain what has been lost and move forward with the progress it has begun until full and totally equal citizenship has been achieved for all.

5

Academic and Mundane Bioethics in Argentina

José Alberto Mainetti

INTRODUCTION

In the Argentinean situation, bioethics is a scholastic endeavor as well as an everyday experience within the culture. Any discussion of bioethics will include both of these perspectives--that of the Latin American intellectual and of the non-academic who meets bioethical dilemmas in everyday life.

The present development of comparative bioethics at an international and transcultural level shows signs of its maturity as it makes its way to universality. We are beginning to see some identity in our differences and unity in our plurality. In a previous paper, "Bioethical Problems in the Developing World: A View from Latin America,"[7] I made a comparative study, through a descriptive, normative, and metaethical analysis, of Western culture in the Anglo-American and Latin American traditions as regards the *ethos* and ethics in biomedicine. Based on this analysis and on my own experience as director of a process involved in institutionalizing bioethics in Argentina, I would like to propose another approach to the "transcultural dimensions of medical ethics." This approach has had three phases over the past twenty years: that of introducing bioethics, of gaining acceptance for its analyses and implications, and of its implementation.

The present international comparative work aims at an exchange of viewpoints concerning foundational topics in bioethics--the concepts, methods, and ends that shape the theory or system of medical ethics--rather than a description of the differences or coincidences in the approaches to and solutions for specific ethical dilemmas in the biomedical context. In substance, this chapter tries to show certain transcultural shapings which have occured when

Western foundations of bioethics have been transplanted to a land which is not its natural, or native one. It has shown us both faces of the coin, the academic and the mundane, or applied; what we have found is that we need to make a new coin in our own system. The academic side of Argentina's bioethical system has been developed and continues to be developed in several ways, each with its own thesis and comparative position regarding applications to the discipline. Such positions are representative of the approach that Latin Americans, in general, and Argentineans, in particular, are taking to ethical questions, and they emphasize the values we consider important for biomedical decisionmaking.

INSTITUTO DE HUMANIDADES MEDICAS
(INSTITUTE OF MEDICAL HUMANITIES)

The Institute of Medical Humanities of the Mainetti Foundation, founded in 1969, is the first institution of its kind in South America entirely devoted to research, documentation, and teaching of those disciplines--particularly the history and philosophy of medicine as it developed in North America and Europe during the seventies. The effects of the revolutionary mentality engendered by this new focus of modern medicine echoed in our institute. This resulted mainly in the establishment of the publishing house Quiron, which has published twenty issues of a journal of the same name since 1970, as well as a series of twenty volumes, books, and texts on various topics. The institute has also organized many national and international meetings on medical humanities and bioethics.[8]

For the institute, the seventies was a period of assimilating the medical humanities of other times and cultures, quite similar to the European experience during which it developed a unique medical humanism. The principal sources in our case were the Spanish school of the history of medicine (P. Lain Entralgo), the German school of medical anthropology (H. Schipperges), and the French school of biological epistemology (G. Canguilhem). This period of assimilation of current bioethical thinking was marked by the growth of personal and institutional relationships with others in the discipline.

The medical humanities movement, partly influenced by Anglo-Saxon philosophy of science, represents a critical difficulty in the use of the traditional scientific paradigm for medical problem-solving, restructuring the paradigm to include medical models based on humanistic, anthropological, holistic, or bio-psycho-social premises. For us, also, the acceptance of the medical humanities indicated difficulties with the inherited scientific medical paradigm for problem-solving in pathology, clinical medicine, and treatment modalities. These new models are part of a philosophy of medicine with three main branches: medical anthropology, medical epistemology, and medical ethics. This is the reason that, from the very beginning, our approach to bioethics has been more theoretical than pragmatic and more principle-based than case-oriented. Nevertheless, we are aware of the advantages and disadvantages of each approach and of the necessary reciprocal complementarity. To express it metaphorically, even caricaturally: medicine today is itself ill; one treatment would be large doses of ethics, and another would be the administering of the essence of humanity.[24]

CATEDRA DE HUMANIDADES MEDICAS
(CHAIR OF MEDICAL HUMANITIES)

In 1980, the Faculty of Medical Sciences of La Plata created the Postgraduate Chair of Medical Humanities, a unique undertaking in Latin America. The University of La Plata thereby became the national and regional academic leader in these disciplines. The chair develops the programs for humanities in medicine, identifies specialized human resources, and achieves national and international interaction by means of its academic extension activities. The latter activities have included the fourth National Conference on the History of Medicine in Argentina, P. Lain Entralgo's visit as doctor honoris causa to the National University of La Plata, and the annual meetings on Medical Humanities and International Symposia of Bioethics.[17]

During the first five years of the chair, Argentina was experiencing the "assimilation stage" of bioethics, thus defining the epistemological and pedagogical aspects of medical ethics as developed in the United States in the sixties. We held our first three international symposia on bioethics, at which were gathered the few national specialists on the subject as well as two well-known representatives from the United States: Tristram Engelhardt and Ronald Bayer.[18] During this period I was able to participate in the tenth Intensive Course of Bioethics (Kennedy Institute of Ethics, Georgetown University, Washington, DC, June 1 to 6, 1984). This experience led to a paper titled, "Foundations of Biomedical Ethics," inspired by my experience in the United States, which was presented at the first National Ethics Conference held in Buenos Aires, Argentina, August 1984.[16]

During this period of theoretical assimilation, bioethics took first place among the medical humanities, becoming an important theory of interdisciplinary synthesis in the systematic philosophy of modern medicine. However, the new philosophical ethics that evolved was primarily analytical and critical. When applied to clinical medicine, this approach conflicts with traditional professional deontology, still widely accepted, which arose from the codified, dogmatic Hippocratic tradition. Consequently, a critical attitude was the general response to the new model of medical ethics, especially the "theory of moral justification" originating at Georgetown and based on the application of principles applied to cases in order to solve conflicts. The alternative has been propelled by a new current in Anglo-American bioethics literature[3] which may be summarized in three major categories:

1. Conceptual: Based on foundations of morals other than the axiomatic or epistemological.

2. Methological: A more empirical, inductive, or intuitive moral reasoning; for example, casuistry as the counterpart of formal or deductive "moral engineering."

3. Applied: *Eupraxis*, as an antonym of *malpraxis*, a focus which calls for a rehabilitation of the professional virtue *ethos*, of moral ideals, and of a therapeutic relationship grounded on doctor-patient *philia* (friendship).

PROGRAMA DE INVESTIGACIONES BIOETICAS
(PROGRAM FOR BIOETHICAL INVESTIGATION)

Since 1985, the Institute and the Chair of Medical Humanities have jointly fostered the Program for Bioethical Investigations (hereafter PIBE). This program consists of an interdisciplinary group of researchers whose projects deal with both the foundations of bioethics and the study of specific topics through systematic and analytical approaches, respectively. From a comparative and transcultural perspective, the PIBE studies the biomedical ethical profile in Argentina, particularly the most significant issues of national concern.[11]

With the PIBE, the next stage of development of bioethics began at individual, group, and institutional levels. This has been termed the "production stage." During this period, the majority of my papers and three books were devoted to theoretical bioethics and its principal issues.[14] The work of the group followed the general direction of the discipline in the treatment of the main topics of bioethical debate in Argentina, such as definition of death, ethics of organ transplantation, beginning of life, the morality of new reproductive technologies, and issues related to AIDS. This stage has been productive in that it has fostered the process of establishing autonomy in the Argentinean bioethical context. Its productivity has also been expressed by the development of a number of official bioethical agencies created around the Center for Bioethics.

At this point, we understand bioethics to be a practical form of philosophy, both as moral and as political philosophy, which challenges medicine to take a new ethical direction. Derived from the terms *bios*, meaning life and *ethiké*, meaning ethics, the discipline is conceptually a synthesis of the advances of science and the mandates of conscience. So the concept of bioethics goes beyond traditional medical ethics, addressing itself to the bioethical crises of the current technological era. This is a moral crisis occurring as a result of these main trends:

- The catastrophic destruction of the environment,
- The great discoveries in biology,
- The technicalization of life.

In response to these, medicine has expressed itself in three innovative ways:

- Covenant-based medical ethics, developed from the Noah-God relationship in the Bible,

- Desire-based medical ethics, developed from the mythological figure of Pygmalion,
- Power medicine, as described by the novelist Knock.

All of these have changed the chimerical face of biomedical ethics.[5] The historical foundation which is the basis for the discipline or, as Nietzsche says, the "genealogy of morals," provides the systematic reasoning underlying the taxonomy of macro, meso, and micro levels and thereby gives order to the larger issues of bioethics. It also gives order to our program of investigation, the projects of which explore the most pressing topics in the country, thereby submitting them to comparative study, both descriptive and conceptual.

The heart of comparative bioethics seems to be the dialogue between those seeking a universal biomedical perspective, those holding traditional values within specific cultures, and those representing mainstream Western culture. Nominally and conceptually bioethics is an offspring of Western culture, characterized by scientific voluntarism or the technological imperative, and libertarian or secular morals. But it is a radical change of the traditional *bios* and *ethos* through manipulation of life and secularization of morals and it is not acceptable from the Latin American perspective or from that of other so-called third world countries. In these countries, technological advances are not implemented and the ethical pluralism which is a result of modern democracy is not present. The Latin American bioethics profile could be defined, *prima facie*, as a "pre-technical," practical, and closed system of morality. It is based on the principle of the holiness of life and the imperatives of natural law that are traditionally supported by Roman Catholic moral theology which has historically maintained prominence in the morality of Latin America.

These traditional values of human nature are based on a particular understanding of human dignity. When making bioethical decisions regarding the proper use of technology for problems of human life, and particularly, for new methods to assist reproduction and dying, these values fashion a Pygmalionic revolution, anthropoplastic or autopoietic.

Catholic moral theology governs policies on abortion and euthanasia, both of which are legally prohibited in the majority of Latin American countries. No public debate or dissenting legislation on the matter has been presented up to now. At a macrobioethical level, one must add to the problems of abortion and euthanasia the problem of the ethics of population control. The Christian perspective, or, more specifically, the Catholic position, insists upon two related aspects which express the tension between private and public morality: limits on contraceptive methods (the rhythm method being the only licit one) and on global population policies. When considered from a perspective that is not Catholic, new technologies which aid reproduction, such as IVF, have led to the development of many subtleties in the bioethics dialogue. And these are very interesting. But in Latin America the Catholic religious justification remains the basis on which bioethical decisions are made. One example of this is the use of whole brain death as a criterion for determining readiness for organ transplantation. This is an honoring of individual human dignity from the perspective mentioned.

CENTRO DE BIOETICA
(CENTER FOR BIOETHICS)

In 1986, with the new installations in the Centro Oncológico de Excelencia (Oncologic Center), the Mainetti Foundation created the National Reference Center for Bioethics (henceforth CENAREBIO). Incorporated into a modern health center--unique in Argentina because of its concept and setting--the CENAREBIO is a kind of laboratory where bioethical studies are taught according to methods developed internationally. These activities have made the center a national and international source of information and documentation.[14]

The second stage of bioethics, that of systematic national development and international exchange, began by putting into practice the pragmatic goals of the center: academic (scientific research and postgraduate teaching), the consultative (clinical ethics committees), and policymaking (public policy recommendations about biomedical dilemmas). At the same time that a national bioethical network is being woven, an international collaborative bridge among the most noted centers of the world is also being built. And prominent bioethicists, such as Sandro Spinsanti, Warren Reich, Hans-Martin Sass, Charles Culver, and Diego Gracia Guillén,[15] have participated in our meetings during November each year.

At the center, bioethics is not only an academic, consultative, and policymaking discipline, but also a culture of civil morality. In fact, bioethics began in the United States to uphold a human right, that of the autonomy of patients in the face of traditional medical paternalism. The introduction of the moral subject in medicine and the participation of the rational and free agent in therapeutic decisions is certainly a historical conquest. The phenomenon on which paternalism is based is a kind of medicalization of life and morality in which health is equal to welfare and this becomes the highest criterion for morality. Responding to this, bioethics with its principles of beneficence, autonomy, and justice has become the most representative body of doctrine for civil morality in the developed world. However, the application of these principles, clinically or legally, presumes an increasingly conflictive set of relations between patient, physician, and society. The situation is not yet like this in Argentina. There is neither major public questioning of medical authority nor much concern about quality of life under the light of the technological imperative of modern medicine. (*Quinlan* is not a well-known case in our media.) Our challenge is to develop our own bioethical culture. We have learned from the experiences of bioethicists around the world and are mindful not to stumble over the same difficulties. We are eager to take advantage of a renewal of values in biomedicine so that we may accomplish a strong social morality during periods of moral crisis.[19]

COMITE HOSPITALARIA DE ETICA
(HOSPITAL ETHICS COMMITTEE)

The Oncology Center Ethics Committee is the first of its type in Argentina. We planned it to be the beginning of a national network of new normative boards in health care similar to those in the United States, which have popped up like mushrooms following a rainstorm. Ours is an interdisciplinary committee: the majority of members are physicians and philosophers working with the aid of a lawyer; there is also an anthropologist and a Catholic priest. The excellent cooperation of hospital staff has made the task of the committee easier. Once a week the ethics board reads and comments on cases, studies precedents of similar cases, and discusses primary bioethical issues such as doctor-patient relationships, patient care, new technologies, experimentation on human subjects, and topics related to death and dying.[13]

For us, the ethics committee is a most fortunate bioethical development, a battle horse in the humanizing crusade for moral medical practice. I see it as having three types of functions as a moral agent:

- Conceptual--because the ethics committee is, or ought to be, an ideal community of communication, and mutual consent, not just the mere locus for strategic of negotiation.
- Methological--because case studies are the basis for practical reasoning in clinical ethics.
- Practical (in the Kantian sense of the word)--because of moral development within the committee of individual prudence and conscience leading to the development of these virtues at an institutional level.[23]

Ours is an oncological hospital. Committee teamwork allows information management with patients, permitted in the traditional Hippocratic *ethos*, which is paternalistic and beneficence-oriented as contrasted with full informed consent--required by the Anglo-American liberal *ethos*, contractualist and autonomist. We may also say there is a contraposition between two ethics, as McIntyre remarked in *After Virtue*.[20] This developed from the classical tradition of virtue and arose out of the modern orientation toward principles, whose proponents were the Mediterraneans and the Anglo-Saxons. For the latter, the emphasis is on autonomy, but the good for patients cannot be reached by honoring this principle alone. It can only be reached within a friendly, reciprocal, doctor-patient relationship. Prioritizing the principle of autonomy over beneficence does not address the patient's dependence, however; it just transfers it from the physician to the system.[21] Nevertheless, medical practice does not change substantially in that the vulnerable patient still brings his or her body and mind (and, in some sense, turns that part of the self over to) the physician, becoming dependent due to the reality of the situation of illness. Ethics committees, whose role in the American health system is to solve clinical dilemmas according to a consultative model that combines clinical and legal procedures, informed consent, and freedom of choice, would do well to be aware of this dependence during illness.[14] The true function of ethics committees is not the easy solving of problems but the proper questioning of them; and this activity should be directed to the development of moral guidelines rather than the legal resolution on conflicts.

COMISION NACIONAL DE BIOETICA
(NATIONAL COMMISSION OF BIOETHICS)

In November 1989, the Presidente Secretariat of Science and Technology requested that our center create a National Commission of Bioethics. Though we had previously engaged in similar conversations with provincial and national members of the legislative power, we believed the Secretariat of Science and Technology to be the most suitable jurisdiction for bioethical policies in the country. The statutary outline submitted to the State Secretariat contained the following ten items: foundations, antecedents, definition, concept, jurisdiction, goals, composition, functions, and programs.

The present scientific and technologic biomedical advances, with their increasing social, ethical, and legal implications, shape a totally new bioethical context, one that is both biological and cultural. Its management calls for the highest political responsibility of our time. National commissions of bioethics are a way for public powers to face the challenge of a new ethics of life in developed societies because governments must make political decisions about issues that require public debate, and expert advice and recommendations. The suitability of public policy recommendations by bioethics commissions--when they are authentically reflective and mediate between community sensibility and state intervention--relies on teamwork, or "commissional bioethics" as a model of civil morality because of its pluralistic consensus and democratic solution of the normative questions in biomedicine. To be a member of a political commission then, is the fulfillment of the main responsibility for a bioethicist, who must never fall into "moral malpraxis." Comparative bioethical studies which contemplate the experience of other countries while at the same time considering the state of the discipline in our own, initially help this exercise.[1]

Some features of the Argentinean bioethical profile support the jurisdiction of the Secretariat of Science and Technology as an advisory board on such policies in our country. With the restoration of democracy in 1983, practical philosophy, that is, philosophical reflection on ethics and politics, became fashionable. Ideological pluralism and the necessity of consensus returned in a lively way to public debate about human rights, war, and peace.[10] This was succeeded by the movement toward scientific ethics, an ethics which is increasingly related, because of its foundations and its applications, to a science whose value-neutrality is being questioned.[2]

Only a couple of events that transpired publicly affected the morality of the Argentinean scientific community: the crotoxina case--involving an experimental, unauthorized drug, given to patients with cancer, and the "Azul episode"--a clandestine experiment with a recombinant virus.[9] Both events may be considered as the awakening of a bioethical culture in the American sense, that is to say, a movement of public interest especially directed to the recognition of a patient's right to make decisions about his or her own body. Whereas the Anglo-Saxon jurisprudence system leaves the solving of those bioethical conflicts in the hands of common law, Latin American judicial reasoning prefers to foresee and formulate relevant constitutional legislation (statutory law). In sum, because of our political tradition, the executive via offers better possibilities than the judicial or the legislative (as it began in Latin America) for bioethics to become biolaw and gain a place in civil life.

ESCUELA LATINOAMERICANA DE BIOETICA
(LATIN AMERICAN SCHOOL OF BIOETHICS)

The Latin American School of Bioethics (henceforth ELABE) of the Mainetti Foundation is a project with the goal of education in bioethical issues and consequent influence on cultural norms and public policy. Until now, there has been no professional or governmental research, no educational program, and no health policy program. Our goal is to prepare bioethicists to develop bioethics programs in their native countries, and to establish a forum of cultural and scientific exchange in the regions. A pioneer in the specialty, ELABE is supported by the National University of La Plata which is an accredited Latin American University, and the Panamerican Sanitary Bureau, which is responsible for the promotion of bioethical studies in Latin America and the Caribbean.[11]

ELABE, in its formation stage, centered its activity on an International Course of Bioethics (420 hours) which was repeated during its first three years (1990-92) from September to November. The course has been chaired by prominent professors from the leading international centers of the discipline (Kennedy Institute, Hastings Center, and other university centers such as the Dartmouth Medical School, Baylor College, and the Cleveland Clinic Foundation, together with other European and Latin American schools). At the end of those three years, the organizational experience, an increased understanding of regional needs, and the availability of qualified bioethicists, allowed us to finally institutionalize the school.[12]

ELABE is an ambitious project which aims at transcultural and international cooperation in bioethics. It pursues a definition of bioethical philosophy from the Latin American perspective which is complementary to that of the Anglo-American. On one hand, let us say the "mundane," or "applied," ELABE is attempting to encourage regional integration and application of bioethical developments. On the other hand, that of the "academic," the aim is to form an alternative bioethics different from that developed out of the traditional individualistic Anglo-American perspective. This new bioethics will emphasize the analysis of social dimensions of medicine, a focus left unattended by the Western paradigm of health care. In industrialized countries bioethical issues have been pre-eminently fashioned by high technology medicine: the allocation and application of procedures related to intensive care, dialysis, transplants, reproductive technologies, and others have been generators of many moral dilemmas. On the contrary, the center of gravity for a bioethical thought truly fruitful for Latin America can be found in a consideration of the deficient provision and significant maldistribution of health care in underdeveloped countries and in the role of the government regarding individuals and populations.

In developed countries bioethical change is characterized by technicalization of life processes and by moral secularization. In developing countries this bioethical perspective is hued by a pretechnical notion of *bios*, and a communitarian notion of *ethos*. In such a case, we ought to contrast the neologism "bioethics," which has come to mean a synthesis of liberal ethics and technological processes affecting life, with the term "hygienomia," meaning a synthesis of authentic health and common morality: they are the two main faces of bioethics, the ethics of individual and of collective human life.[1]

CONCLUSION

In summary, this presentation of the process of the institutionalization of bioethics in Argentina tries to depict some transcultural shapings of the discipline which may be useful as references in a comparative discussion of specific issues in medical ethics.

I propose that there are six premises about these transcultural models of bioethics:

1. As a philosophy of medicine--its theoretical and foundational basis contrasts with that of pragmatism and libertarianism.
2. As a medical ethics--its conceptual, methological, and practical models are together an alternative to that which is solely a principle-based ethics.
3. As a health culture--it is a traditional paternalist physician *ethos* opposed to the notion autonomy as a civil right.
4. As a method of assistance--it can be applied by the institution of two hospital ethics committees, one to ask moral questions and another to give legal answers.
5. As a political endeavor--it is an executive national commission rather than a judicial method or a legislative body for the making of biolaw.
6. As an academic endeavor--it is a Latin American school of health care ethics which complements the Anglo-American form of clinical ethics.

Although there are other individuals and institutions which deserve to be included as representatives of bioethics in Argentina, the modest scene just described would not change substantially. Nevertheless, we can foresee, like other peoples of world, the rapid development of bioethics as the "ethics of life" in an age of technology, and as a challenge to the development of man as a moral being in the anthropoplastic revolution of the "brave new medical world."

The dialogue into which we entered at the Fidia Symposium expresses the new face of humanism represented by bioethics from three distinct perspectives: interdisciplinary, pluralist, and transcultural. It is from such a complete perspective that we may form a lasting cooperative context in which individuals, varying cultures, and new knowledge are part of the same dialogue.

NOTES

1   Bioethics Commissions: International Perspectives. *The Journal of Medicine and Philosophy* 1989;14. See this article to note the coincidence among the recommendation of authors that such commissions be more philosophical and include a greater representation of those with ethical backgrounds.

2   Bunge M. In the work of this author, the founding of the Asociación Argentina de Investigaciones Eticas, and the appearance of the journal *Etica y Ciencia* are eloquent statements of the increasing development of the ethics of science in Argentina.

3   Childress J.F. The Normative Principles of Medical Ethics, In: Veatch R.M. *Medical Ethics, Boston*: Jones and Bartlett Publishers, 1989. This article contains a synopsis of recent critics of the principles and rules model of biomedical ethics. Along the same lines, consult also Toulmin S. and Jonsen A. Defense of casuistry. In: *The Abuse of Cauistry: A History of Moral Reasoning*. Berkeley, California: The University of California Press, 1981. See also works by Piaget and Kohlberg who have developed theories of moral development, and Carol Gilligan (*In a Different Voice*. Cambridge: Harvard University Press, 1982) who has pioneered in issues of gender morality. *The Task Force on Experience as a Source of Bioethics*, directed by Warren Reich and supported by I.H. Page Center for Creative Thinking in Medicine, A Division of the Cleveland Clinic Foundation (Reich, W. Bioethics Paradigm, *Kennedy Institute Newsletter*, 1989;3:4) is another important contribution. A systematic criticism to the principles model is that of K. Danner Clouser and Bernard Gert in their: A Criticism of Principalism, an unpublished manuscript given to me by Charles Culver.

4   Fleetwood T.E., Arnold R.M., Baron R.J. Giving Answers or Raising Questions? The Problematic Role of Institutional Ethics Committees. *Journal of Medical Ethics*, September 1989;15:3;137-142.

5   Mainetti J.A. Bioética Fundamental. In press. A development of these ideas can be found in this text.

6   Mainetti J.A. Bioética: una nueva filosofia de la salud. Boletin Especial de Bioética de la Oficina Sanitaria Panamericana. In press (Mayo-Junio 1990).

7   Mainetti J.A. Bioethical problems in the developing world: a view from Latin America. *Unitas* 1987;60;238-248.

8   Mainetti J.A., ed. *Boletin del Instituto de Humanidades Mëdicas y Centro de*

Bioética, No .1, November 1988 and No. 2 July 1989. Editorial Quiran, La Plata.
9   Mainetti J.A. El caso de la crotoxina: un espectro bioético nacional. In: *Etica y Ciencia*, Invierno, 1988;II:2.
10   Mainetti J.A. *El Conflicto del Médico*. Quiron 1982;13;3-4. On the "missing" and the bioethics of filiation, "the guerrilla" and the War of Malvinas.
11   Mainetti J.A. El Programa de Investigaciones Bioeticas. In: *Introduccion a la Bioética*, 35-41.
12   Mainetti J.A., ed. ELABE: *Programa del Curso de Éspecializacion en Bioética* 1990. La Plata:Quiron, 1990.
13   Mainetti J.A. *Filosofos al Hospital: Los Comités de Etica*. Quiron 1984;15:2; Protocolo de Bochum para la practiva ético-médica. Zentrum fur Medizinische Ethik. Bochum:Medizinethische Materialem, Heft 23, 1988. In collaboration with Hans-Martin Sass and Herbert Viefhues.
14   Mainetti J.A. Introduccion a la bioética. La crisis de la razon médica. In: *Introduccion a la Filosofia de la Medicina*, La Plata, Quiron, 1988; Etica Médica:Introduccion historica, La Plata:Quiron, 1989. Consult this reference for more information about the Center for Bioethics and the Oncological Center for Excellence.
15   Mainetti J.A., ed. II y III Jornadas de Humanidades Médicas y Simposio Internacional de Bioética, La Plata:Quiron, 1988; IV y V Jornadas de Humanidades Médicas y Simposio Internacional de Bioética, La Plata:Quiron, 1989.
16   Mainetti J.A. La fundamentacion de la ética biomédica. In: *Introduccion a la Bioética*, 7-13.
17   Mainetti J.A. *Leccion Inaugural del Catedra de Humanidades Médicas*. Quiron 1980;11:2;65-73.
18   Mainetti J.A. Nuestros estudios bioéticos en quince anos de Humanidades Médicas. In: *Introduccion a la Bioética*, La Plata:Editorial Quiron, 1987, 28-34.
19   Mainetti J.A. SIDA: la crisis de la salud y la moral publicas, Quiron 1988;19:1. AIDS is the "bioethics disease" by antonomasia and it is the paradigmatic issue for transcultural analysis.
20   McIntyre A. After Virtue, Notre Dame: University of Notre Dame Press, 1983.
21   Pellegrino E.D., Mc Elhinney T., 1981. *Teaching Ethics, The Humanities, and Human Values in Medical Schools: A Ten Year Overview*. Washington, DC: The Society for Health and Human Values; Fox DM. Who We Are: The Political Origins of the Medical Humanities. Theoretical Medicine 1985;6;327-342. Our medical humanities model coincided notably with one of the first and more important anthologies on the subject, that edited by Chester R. Burns and Tristram Englehardt in The Texas Report on Biology and Medicine 1974;32:1, titled *The Humanities in Medicine*. Another significant encounter between Anglo-American and Hispanic American medical humanities was the IXth Interdisciplinary Symposium of Philosophy and Medicine, chaired by E. Pellegrino and P. Lain Entralgo in Madrid, March 1979. At this symposium devoted to the ethics of diagnosis, I delivered the lecture: Embodiment, Pathology and

Diagnosis, later published in *Ethics of Diagnosis*. Dordrecht: D. Reidel and further submitted for publication.

22 Pellegrino E.D., Thomasma D.C. *For the Patient's Good. The Restoration of Beneficence in Health Care*. New York: Oxford University Press, 1988. According to Mark Siegler's thesis, the millenary "age of paternalism" was succeeded in the United States after 1985 by "the age of autonomy," which, in turn, has been replaced by "the age of beaurocratic parsimony" introduced in 1983 by Diagnostic-Related-Groups for Medicare and Medicaid (p. 28)

23 Tealdi J.C., Mainetti J.A. Los comites hospitalarios de etica. *Boletin Especial de Bioética de la Oficina Sanitaria Panamericana. In press (Mayo-Junio, 1990).*

24 Thomasma D.C. The Philosophy of Medicine in Europe. *Theoretical Medicine*, 1985;6:1. On the contrast between the European and North American mentality in medical philosophy. Though this issue inexcusably lacks a reference about the philosophy of medicine in Spain, the latter belongs to the same European tradition and we acknowledge it as such.

6

Islamic Basis for Biomedical Ethics

Hassan Hathout

INTRODUCTION

As a Muslim living in the West, I realize that knowledge about Islam is tremendously lacking as well as riddled with misconceptions. For a chapter dealing with an Islamic issue to be meaningful, it is necessary to devote some space to brief the reader about Islam, even in the most general terms, so as to be able to cope with further data and put them in proper perspective. Some Islamic ideas seem to be out of place when the current Western concept of the word "religion" is applied, and only a prior understanding of the message, scope, and general anatomy of Islam can put them in their logical context. It is our conviction therefore that a general outline of Islam, and perhaps a description of where it stands in relation to its predecessors, Judaism and Christianity, should be the foundation upon which to base such specific and seemingly isolated issues as the Islamic foundations of biomedical ethics.

Islam is the third of the monotheistic religions commonly referred to as the Abrahamic religions, following Judaism and Christianity. The three principal figures of these religions share the ancestry of Abraham: Moses and Jesus through his son Isaac, and Mohammad through his son Ismail. They all embrace the Abrahamic creed of belief in God (Allah in Arabic, Yahweh in Hebrew) and His oneness. Uniquely, Islam recognizes the other two religions and proclaims itself as the last link of the long chain of God-sent messages. The book of Islam is the Quran, which Muslims believe is the record of God's very words conveyed to Mohammad by the Angel Gabriel. It was revealed in short passages over the span of twenty-three years as occasion arose, and as soon as Mohammad uttered it, it was memorized by heart as well as written down, so that its original text remains intact to the letter. The Quran addresses those who believe in it saying: "Say ye, we believe in God and the revelation given to us, and to Abraham, Ismail, Isaac, Jacob and the Tribes, and that given to Moses and Jesus, and that given the Prophets from their Lord, we make no discrimination between one and another of them, and to Him we are submitters (meaning Muslims) [2:136]." This unity in God and unity in faith is reiterated in various passages of the Quran, such as: "The same religion has He established for you as that which He enjoined on Noah, that which We revealed unto thee, and that which We enjoined on Abraham, Moses and Jesus, namely that you should remain steadfast in Religion and make no divisions therein [42:13]."

It is no wonder therefore that the commonalties between the three religions are so great, a fact extensively unknown, especially regarding Islam. The moral codes of the three religions practically--if not literally--coincide. Islam holds Jews and Christians in special regard, and gives them the honorary title of "the People of the Books," being fellow believers in the One God and the recipients of the messages of the Torah and the Ingeel respectively.

And yet it is as important to identify the differences between Jews and Christians as it is to know the commonalities, so that mutual stands can be based on facts and not on sweeping stereotypes, well entrenched over many centuries, but the product of distortion and emotionalism. The fact that neither Jews nor Christians recognize Islam as a God-sent religion can be set aside by the response that the main doctrinal differences between Islam and both the followers of Judaism and Christianity are not differences with what Moses and Jesus taught, but with later interpretations or conceptualizations by their followers.

With their Jewish cousins, Muslims disagree on the concept of the Chosen People. The Quran is full of praise of the Children of Israel who in their time were the only segment of humanity professing belief in God and His oneness; but the criterion for judging Muslims is obedience to God and observation of His guidance, and not loyalty to a special selection of leaders qualifying by lineage or otherwise. The Quran declares: "Ye mankind: We have created you from a single pair, a male and a female, and made nations and tribes out of you so that you may get to know and cherish one another, and not that you may despise one another, verily the best of you in the sight of God are the most righteous [49:13]."

The Quran also rebukes the Israelites for certain mutinous attitudes against their prophets, Moses and others [22:91]. A major difference, of course, is in regard to Jesus of Nazareth. Whereas the Jews are still awaiting the Messiah while rejecting Jesus and refuting his virgin birth, the Quran describes Jesus as a genuine messenger from God, a Spirit who He bestowed on Mary. God chose her, purified her, and willed that she give birth to Jesus without being "touched" by a human being. "And (remember) her who guarded her chastity. We breathed into her of Our Spirit and We made her and her son a sign for all people [22:91]."

But it is also on the identity of Jesus that Islam holds a major difference with Christians. In Islam Jesus was miraculously created by God without a father, and he was neither divine nor God's son. The concept of the Trinity, decreed to be the creed of the Roman Empire by the Council of Nicea in 325 AD, is not acceptable to Islam. Nor is the concept of vicarious atonement to redeem mankind, for every person is responsible for his or her own individual deeds. God's forgive-ness and mercy can be approached by personal repentance without bloodshed or even intercession between human beings and their Creator; hence, there is no clergy and no church in Islam. Original sin is not inheritable, the original sinners--Adam and Eve--had been forgiven before Adam was chosen to prophethood and sent to earth, and every human being is therefore born in purity.

It is fortunate that, at the same time Islam identifies these doctrinal differences, it prescribes a policy of friendliness and justice towards the People of the Book to the extent that a Muslim may marry one of their women and he is never permitted to pressure her into becoming Muslim and is indeed instructed to ensure her right of worship in her own way.

THE *SHARI'A*

Beside confirming the moral code of its predecessors, Islam adds the framework of a total legal system to regulate and organize various aspects of human activities. Law is a human necessity, and morals alone are not enough for actual government of society nor can they abound in a legal vacuum. This total system of Islam is called the *Shari'a*, and although comprehensive, only a few rulings in it are fixed. It represents outlines which allow for flexibility and for new rulings to be evolved to suit new circumstances in changing times and places, but always within the general framework.

This explains why the concept of separation of church and state does not pertain in Islam. On the one hand the state is within the concern of *Shari'a*, and, on the other, there is no church. There is no theocratic government, and an ideal Islamic government according to the *Shari'a* would have probably been very similar to a standard Western democracy, but with the Quran as its constitution, which means that God shall neither be vetoed nor outvoted. The flexibility of the *Shari'a* has led to the accumulation over the ages of a wealth of laws and rulings collectively called *Fiqh* or *Islamic Jurisprudence*. Juridical schools appeared, with a wide spectrum of interpretations even within the same school. Imam Shafie (died 204 H/819 AD), the founder of one of the major juridical schools or *madhabs*, wrote a second version of his *madhab* when he moved from Baghdad to Cairo, where he found new circumstances and social customs. Before him, Omar, the second caliph, was asked about the same issue and gave different rulings on two successive years, saying: we ruled upon what we then knew and we rule upon what we now know. The religion remains the same, and rulings specifically mentioned in the Quran are constant and these are only few.

Otherwise, it is up to human thinking to devise new rulings for new situations as long as there is no conflict with the spirit of the religion or trespassing outside the goals of the *Shari'a*. It is upon the knowledge and regard of these that the relevant rulings on various issues should be sought: the Islamic basis for biomedical ethics being no exception.

THE SOURCES OF THE *SHARI'A*

There are four principal sources of the *Shari'a*, as well as other subsidiary ones. A brief account of these will be given, starting with the principal sources which are the Quran, The Tradition of the Prophet, The Universal Consensus of Scholars, and Analogy.

1. The Quran. This is the record of the direct and very words of God conveyed by the Angel Gabriel to the Prophet Mohammad. A translation of the Quran is not called Quran since it will not be an exact record of the very words of God, however accurate that translation may be. Things that God gave as inspiration to the Prophet and which the Prophet then expressed in his own words are not Quran. The Quran was revealed over a period of twenty-three years in short segments that were immediately memorized by heart as well as written down, so that the Quran is preserved to the letter. The rearrangement of these segments in the order presented by the book called the *Mos'haf* (the Quran in one book) with 114 *suras,* each with a variable number of verses, was finalized in the life of the Prophet after the whole Quran was revealed upon instructions brought by the Angel Gabriel. The Quran comprises three kinds of rulings: those pertaining to basic creed and belief, those denoting the moral code, and those concerned with practices. The latter comprise two categories: practices of worship that regulate immediate relations with God, and practices of human relationships at the individual, family, social, national and international levels. Whereas creed and belief rulings are specific and detailed, those relating to human relationships give --with few exceptions--broad outlines and general principles, allowing flexibility for the jurisprudence to deduce legislation to suit different times and environments in the multiple spheres of private affairs law, family laws, civil law, penal law, constitutional law, military law, economic law, and international law. The Quran is the primary and ultimate source of the *Shari'a*.

2. The Tradition of Prophet Mohammad *(Sunna)*. This comprises what the Prophet said, did, or approved. Verbal Tradition includes *ahadith* (singular: *hadith*) or sayings of the Prophet. That the Tradition is a principal source of legislation is emphasized by the Quran itself:

Say obey God and His Apostle [3:32].

So establish prayer and give charity and obey the Apostle that you may receive mercy [24:56].

He who obeys the Apostle obeys God [4:80].

It is not befitting for a believer, man or woman, when a matter has been decided by God and His Apostle to have any option about their decision: if any one disobeys God and His Apostle he is indeed on a clearly wrong path [33:36].

The *Sunna* complements the Quran, or explains it, filling in some information on issues that the Quran mentioned without detail and referring to matters not mentioned in the Quran. The science of authentication of the Prophet's sayings is one of the most exhaustive and precise branches of the science of history. The role of *Sunna* in legislation is second to that of the Quran.

3. Consensus. This is the unanimous convergence of the opinions on one ruling on a certain issue of all qualified religious scholars of the Muslim nation (at a single point in time) since the death of the Prophet. It represents unanimity of the nation as represented by its scholars, in the light of the saying of the Prophet: "My nation will never be unanimously in error." If the case under consideration has a relevant ruling in the Quran or *Sunna* then resort to the seeking of Consensus would be superfluous. On the other hand, it is difficult to imagine that unanimity would be attained unless the scholars have strong evidence supporting their ruling.

4. Analogy. This is a means of reasoning which applies to a situation not specifically mentioned in the Quran or *Hadith*, but which can be equated to one that has a ruling from the Quran and/or the *Sunna*, since they both have the same reason for that ruling. An example is the prohibition of alcoholic beverages since they dim and confuse the mind. Although drugs like cocaine and heroin have no mention in the Quran or *Hadith*, the same ruling--by analogy--applies to them because they share the reason for prohibition. Analogy is based on legitimate, honest reasoning and was recommended by the Quran and the Prophet for situations, not previously specified by Quran or *Sunna*.

The remaining sources of the *Shari'a*--as basis for legislation--are subsidiary to the aforementioned ones and will be only briefly described.

5. Istihsan. This means a legitimate exception to a ruling in a particular situation. It is not likely to be the most obvious or the most popular.

6. Public welfare. This concerns issues without positive or negative rulings but which relate to a public function such as the building of hospitals, schools, milling of money, etc.

7. Social custom and culture. This includes that which does not conflict with the essence or the text of the *Shari'a*.

8. Continuity of status quo. This is the continuance of pre-existing situations not ruled against by the *Shari'a*. By nature, everything remains lawful unless specifically prohibited.
9. Rulings of previous God-sent religions. These are to be followed unless abrogated or replaced by Islam's rulings.
10. Authentic opinions of the close companions of the Prophet, who are the direct graduates of his lifelong teaching. These are to be given consideration, although they are not absolutely binding.

THE GOALS OF THE *SHARI'A*

The overall goal of the *Shari'a* is the fulfillment of the welfare of the people by ensuring the satisfaction of their needs, which are technically categorized as indispensable needs, basic needs, and complementary needs, in that order of significance. Each category has its set of rulings while maintaining the order of priority, so that a ruling that aims at a complementary need should not conflict with one addressing a basic need, and a ruling regarding a basic need should not conflict with one regarding an indispensable need. Indispensable needs are those without which human life would be unbearable or chaotic. There are five indispensable needs, namely, the preservation of self (life, health, procreation, nourishment, curing illness, hygiene, etc.); mind (psychological health, relief from stress, avoiding alcohol and drugs, etc.); religion (faith, worship, prayers, fasting, pilgrimage, almsgiving, morality and ethics, etc.); ownership (sanctity of private ownership, legitimate pursuits of wealth, contracts, legitimate commercial relationships, prohibition of stealth, fraud and usury, social functions of capital, etc.); and honor (chastity, prohibition of adultery and sexual offense, marriage and family laws, social conduct, combating moral pollution, etc.). Each of these is covered by a complete set of moral injunctions as well as prescribed laws.

The same applies for ordinary needs (the bulk of the civil and commercial laws) and complementary needs that are meant to improve life, enhance its quality, and augment its enjoyment. It is beyond the scope of this chapter to pursue the rulings specific to each of these needs, for that would be the concern of a book on Islamic jurisprudence. It might be opportune, however, to select some principles incorporated in the *Shari'a* that have a bearing on our discussion of biomedical ethics. These principles guide actions in the following categories:

1. The Role of Mankind in the Universe

Man is God's vicegerent on earth: "Behold, thy Lord said to the angels: I will create a vice regent on earth [2:30]."

Man is therefore entrusted with this planet to manage it in the way consistent with the prescribed plan of the Creator. Man was given both knowledge and guidance towards this goal, as well as the freedom of choice which is the basis of human accountability. The vicegerency entails man's endowment with a creative mind, as well as a full mandate to make conscious use of the nature that surrounds him and is within him: "And He has made subservient to you as from Himself all that is in the heavens and on earth [45:13]." The human race therefore is fully free to harness and manipulate nature in whatever way that ensures fulfillment of the goals of the *Shari'a*.

2. Changing God's Creation

This refers to a verse in the Quran, with a story behind it that is better from the beginning. We have already referred to the sin of Adam and Eve, to their repentance, and to their forgiveness by God and subsequent choice for God's vice regency on earth. When the devil (Satan) saw the change of events in favor of Adam and Eve, whom he had meant to misguide, the devil did not despair, but instead asked God for a second chance to pursue members of the human community on earth and put them to the test again. God granted the request, but said He would provide them with guidance which would immunize them against the devil's temptations. This guidance would protect all except those who willfully reject it in favor of Satan's temptations. The Quran quotes the rebellious Satan, in an expression of his plans to lead mankind astray, addressing God about mankind: "Verily of thy subjects I shall most certainly take my due share, and shall lead them astray, and fill them with vain desires. And I shall command them so that they cut off the ears of cattle (in idolatrous sacrifice), and I shall command them and they will change God's creation." The verse then continues: "But all who take Satan rather than God for their master do indeed --most clearly--lose all. He (Satan) holds out promises to them and fills them with vain desires, yet whatever Satan promises them is but meant to delude the mind [4:119]."

The expression "changing God's creation" in answer to Satan's lure has commanded attention and generated debate between scholars over the ages. In earlier times it was debated whether the sin of changing God's creation should apply even to simple, domestic cosmetic improvements as well as to cosmetic (and therefore, nonessential) surgical procedures and other types of surgery. An application in vogue nowadays is surgical sexual conversion of male to female and vice versa. This is a practice that has been condemned by Moslem scholars unless it is corrective surgery indicated by a congenital malformation and the purpose is to restore the true sexual identity.

Recently, the development of genetic engineering technology has spurred scholars to evaluate it under the light of this Quranic verse, and the subject is really inviting. After all, has not genetic engineering gone beyond mere change to the capability of producing new creatures hitherto unknown in the order of creation? Fortunately, however, the mainstream of scholars are of the opinion that the application of this Quranic verse should not be carried too far, in case it might obstruct the goals of the *Shari'a* by denying people their indispensable and other needs. Overzealous application could conflict with many forms of therapeutic surgery including appendectomy, tonsillectomy, tumor removal, and other forms of treatment that may be lifesaving and life-enhancing although they entail a change in God's creation. In the same token, genetic engineering utilizing recombinant DNA techniques in order to prevent or cure serious disease should be commended. Other aspects of genetic engineering, however, seem to be more complex and should be given more scrutiny, as we will mention later.

3. The Rule that Necessities Overrule Prohibitions

If something is prohibited by the *Shari'a* but under certain conditions it becomes necessary, for example to preserve life or cure illness, then the prohibition is waived for as long as is necessary. A person facing starvation is permitted to eat unlawful food if only unlawful food is available (e.g., pig meat, which is banned by Judaism and Islam and was made lawful to Christians by Paul and not by Christ). A sick person is exempted from fasting during (the fasting month of) Ramadan, but only for the period he is sick. As the situation of special necessity comes to an end, the prohibition applies again, in observance of yet another rule stating: Necessity is observed only as long as it is a necessity.

4. Choice of the Lesser of Two Harms

If only two options are available, both of which are prohibited or harmful, then it becomes lawful to choose the lesser of the two evils in order to obviate the more serious one. Taking a heart from a cadaver for transplantation is better than leaving the recipient to die. Sacrificing a pregnancy by abortion becomes lawful if the continuation of pregnancy threatens the life of the mother.

5. Repelling Harm Takes Priority Over Retaining Benefits

Exercising rights of ownership may have to be curbed if it entails harm to others. The public health rules of isolation and quarantine are given priority over personal freedoms. Prophet Mohammad said: "If you are going to a city where there is pestilence, then don't enter it. If you are already in it, then don't go out." This rule is further complemented by another rule stating: Personal inconvenience is to be endured in order to obviate public harm.

The Summary Rule: Wherever Welfare Goes, There Goes the Law of God

This is the summary rule for issues not mentioned in the Quran or *Sunna* and which do not lend themselves easily to intelligent reasoning by analogy or the unanimity of all scholars of the Muslim nation in a certain era. Whatever is found to be in the best interests of the nation, provided it does not conflict with the essence of religion or the statutes of the *Shari'a*, can confidently be legislated.

THE SHARI'A AND SCIENCE

1. The *Shari'a* and Scientific Research

The first word revealed in the Quran is "read": "Read in the name of your Lord who created. Created man out of a clot like a leach. Read that your Lord is the most Bountiful, who taught with the pen, taught man what man knew not [96:1-5]. "Mohammad decreed that "the pursuit of knowledge is a command for every Muslim man or woman" and ordained its pursuit "even if one had to travel to China," the furthest of lands known at that time. In order to appreciate the Creator by looking into His creation, the Quran challenges the human mind to think and ponder and be inquisitive: "We will show them Our signs in the horizons and in their own selves until it becomes manifest to them that this is the truth [41:53]." "Say: are those equal, those who know and those who do not know [39:9]?" It recommends the prayer: "Say: O my Lord . . . advance me in knowledge [20:116]." The Quran reminds man of his endowment by which can be gained knowledge, and rebukes those who remain idle, "who have hearts (minds) with which they fail to grasp the truth, and eyes with which they fail to see, and ears with which they fail to hear. Those are like cattle--nay, they are even less conscious of the right way: it is they, they who are the (truly) heedless [7:179]."

What we call scientific research now is called, in juridical terminology, the "uncovering of God's tradition in His creation" by discovering the laws of nature. To reveal these laws is considered a religious duty of mankind. Mohammad said: "The scholar's ink is as honorable as the martyr's blood," and taught that the angels "lower their wings in respect of him who seeks knowledge." It was no wonder then that the rise of Islam was associated with a mighty civilization which excelled in all walks of science. The early years of this civilization witnessed a great translation movement that preserved the Greek heritage which had been actively sought and destroyed by the Baselei emperors at the behest of the Church on the pretext of its paganism. It was from their Arabic translations that Europe later received the Greek books. During the Islamic era, Muslim, Christian, and Jew in the Muslim Empire had the opportunity to fully unfold their academic potentials. Europe's experience of the religious hierarchy was that it had obstructed the progress of science and branded it as godless. This no doubt was the reason for the later separation of church and state, a practice which never appeared in Islam. Scientific research is fully protected by the *Shari'a* and, as there is no church hierarchy, there was no mechanism for censure. At no time was it felt that the emancipation of academic pursuit necessitated or resulted from a dichotomy between science and religion.

Since a divorce between science and religion never occurred in Islam, scientists followed the admonitions and prohibitions of the *Shari'a* in their methodology and heeded the *Shari'a* in promulgating their ethics. A modern illustrative example, which is by no means new in content but rather in phraseology, is the *Islamic Code of Medical Ethics*. Endorsed by many Muslim countries this code was issued by the International Organization of Islamic Medicine (later called Islamic Organization of Medical Sciences) in 1981.[2] It is perhaps opportune to quote from it the following articles relevant to this discussion:

● There is no censorship in Islam on scientific research, be it academic--to reveal the signs of God in His creation, or applied--to aim at the solution of a particular problem.

● Freedom of scientific research shall not entail the subjugation of man by coercing him or subjecting him to definite or probable harm, by withholding treatment for his medical needs, by defrauding him or by exploiting his vulnerability due to material needs.

● The methodology of scientific research and the applications resultant therefrom shall not entail the commission of any sin prohibited by Islam such as fornication, the confounding of genealogy, or deforming or tampering with the essence of the human personality including the freedom and capability to bear responsibility.

● The guiding rule in unprecedented matters falling under no extant text or law is the Islamic dictum: Wherever welfare of the people is found, there exists the law of God.

These and other articles might seem ordinary except that each and every one of them is directly derived from a verse in the Quran or a *Hadith* of the Prophet, not including the last which rests on clear evidence from the *Shari'a*.

2. The *Shari'a* and Medicine

The concept of "cause and effect" is well understood by Islam. Several rulings of the *Shari'a* aim at preserving health and enjoin the seeking of treatment if health is afflicted. Prophet Mohammad said: "Your body has a right over you," and ordered: "Seek treatment: Oh subjects of God . . . for God has created a remedy for every ailment, some known and some not." In his words, "the strong faithful (person) is better than the weak one, and there is goodness in both." Jurists are unanimous in ruling that "medicine" is a *Fardh Kifaya* in every community (a religious duty from which the whole community is exempted if it is undertaken by some). Only the one who has the necessary training is allowed to practice medicine, for the Prophet said "whoever practices medicine and is not known to have acquired its knowledge is liable" (to pay compensation). The doctor-patient contract is a commitment of deed but not of final result . . . so that if the doctor is well-qualified and has dispensed treatment on sound grounds, and if there is no evidence of negligence, then he or she would be in the clear if the desired result is not achieved.

The *Shari'a* is replete with rulings of direct relevance to health issues, and some of these are integral to acts of worship. Ablution is necessary before performing prayers, and entails the washing of the face (and mouth and nostrils), hands and forearms, and feet several times a day. Mohammad taught: "God is beautiful and loves beauty, clean and loves cleanliness." The Prophet prescribed a sort of toothbrush made of a frayed out branchlet of a tree called "sewak." Ritual bathing is mandatory before certain activities (after menstruation, intercourse, etc.), and perineal hygiene is emphasized.

Certain acts of worship might be waived for health reasons, pregnancy, lactation, or menstruation. Eating habits are tempered. "The worst vessel for the Son of Adam to fill is his stomach . . . more appropriately he should assign one third for his food, one third for his drink and one third for the comfort of his breathing," to quote the Prophet Mohammad. Certain foods are unlawful, such as pig meat and the meat of animals having died without proper slaughter. Protection of the mind from alcohol and stupefying drugs is mandatory and these are strictly prohibited in any quantity. Reference has already been made to the basis for isolation and quarantine. Care of the environment is a religious duty. This is illustrated in many *hadiths* of the Prophet, such as, "To remove dirt from the pathway of people is a charity" and "Beware of the three cursed deeds, namely, to put refuse in stagnant water sources, in shady places and in the path trodden by people."

The Prophet enjoined water conservation: "Economize in water even if you are at a flowing river." In respect of wildlife he said: "Whoever kills a sparrow without necessity will face God's punishment for it." An example of the protection of natural parks is his decree: "The Valley of Wajj: its trees shall not be cut, and its game is not to be hunted within the distance of four miles around it . . . and whoever trespasses shall receive punishment." Even during war he would instruct his army: "Do not kill a child or a woman or an old person or a non-belligerent. Do not cut a tree or set fire to date palms, and do not slay an animal except for the purpose of eating. You will come across people in monasteries and convents who are devoted to their worship; leave them in peace to pursue that to which they have devoted themselves."

Before concluding this segment we would like to go back to the *Islamic Code of Medical Ethics*[1] for a few more selected quotations concerning the medical profession.

- *Therapeusis* is a noble profession. God honored it by making it the miracle of Jesus, son of Mary. Abraham, enumerating his Lord's gifts upon him, proclaimed "and if I fall ill He cures me."

- Like all aspects of knowledge, medical knowledge is part of the knowledge of God "who taught man what man never knew."

The study of medicine entails the revelation of God's signs in His creation. "And in yourselves: do you not see [51:21]?" The practice of medicine brings God's mercy to His subjects. Medical practice is therefore an act of worship and charity in addition to being a means of making a living.

- But God's mercy is as accessible to all people, including those who are good and evil, virtuous and vicious and friend and foe, as are the rays of His sun, the comfort of His breeze, the coolness of His water and the bounty of His provision. It is upon this basis that the medical profession must operate, along the single track of God's mercy, never adversarial and never punitive, never taking justice as its goal but rather mercy, in all situations and circumstances.

- In this respect the medical profession is unique. It shall never yield to social pressures motivated by enmity or feud--be it personal, political or military. Enlightened statesmanship will do good by preserving the integrity of the medical profession and protecting its position, keeping it beyond enmity or hostility.

- The preservation of man's life should also include the utmost regard for his dignity, feelings, vulnerability, and the privacy of his sentiments and body parts.

- Health is a basic human necessity and not a matter of luxury. A patient should not be denied services, even if he or she cannot afford the fee.

- The natural prophylaxis against some diseases rests in the revival of such religious values as chastity, purity, self-restraint and refraining from advertently or inadvertently inflicting harm on self or others. To preach these values is "preventive medicine" and therefore lies within the jurisdiction and obligation of the medical profession. (This is a departure from the dictum, widely proclaimed in many communities, that a doctor should not moralize.)

SOME BIOETHICAL APPLICATIONS OF *SHARI'A*

The regard for life has led to a view restricting abortion unless the continuation of pregnancy poses a threat to the mother's life. This was the consensus of a recent conference on human life held in 1985 by the Islamic Organization of Medical Sciences (IOMS).[2] The restrictions, in effect, reversed the opinions of earlier scholars who, for centuries, have maintained that life started between seven and sixteen weeks of pregnancy. Suicide and euthanasia for any reason are also absolutely rejected, and there is a clear warning by the Prophet Mohammad against escaping hardship by taking life.[1]

The protection of life entails the protection and promotion of health by adopting lifestyles conducive to physical and psychological health and avoiding those that lead to harm, as exemplified by the Quranic injunction: "Don't let your own hands throw you into destruction," [2:195] and the Prophet's instruction: "Harm and harming are not of Islam." These teachings are further detailed by his many sayings which are guides for habits and styles of life. In the case of illness, seeking medical treatment becomes mandatory according to the Prophet's ruling, since "for every illness God created He created a remedy--whether yet known or unknown."

When treatment, however, carries no prospect of cure, it ceases to be mandatory. Heroic measures and measures that are actually prolonging the dying process rather than promoting life, may then be given up, but no action should be taken to actively bring about death. Pain and suffering must be alleviated physically (by medication), as well as psychologically. Patience is a great virtue in Islam, generously rewarded by God, and the Prophet says, "When someone suffers (from an illness) God discards his sins as the tree sheds its leaves." Death is the crowning of life, and as one exits from this life he enters the lasting hereafter, looking forward to God's mercy: "O (thou) soul,in (complete) rest and satisfaction, come back to thy Lord well pleased and well pleasing unto Him, enter then among my devotees, and enter My heaven [89:27-30]."

The definition of the moment of death has acquired significance in relation both to removal of life support measures and to procurement of vital organs for transplantation. The certain death of the whole brain, including the brain stem, has been accepted as a criterion for death, by analogy with the older juridical rule called "the status of the slain." If a person were to stab another, eviscerating the victim, it would be considered a fatal injury. If a further aggressor were to complete the killing, it would still be the first who would be charged with murder, but the second with assaulting the cadaver. This old ruling has been changed because intestinal injury can now be dealt with surgically, and brain stem death has been recognized as the fatal situation. But the point is the same.[2] Organ donation from the living is considered a great charity according to the Quranic saying: "And if anyone saved a life, it would be as if he saved the whole people [5:35]." Procurement of organs from a cadaver for transplantation is permitted, observing due process, according to the juridical rule of the choice of the lesser of two evils, since desecrating the dead body by cutting is of lower priority than saving the life of the patient.[3] A cadaver may be kept on life support for some time to preserve the suitability of the needed organ for transplantation.

In the area of reproduction, reference has already been made to abortion, although family planning by contraception judiciously used, free of harm, and not entailing the taking of life, is permitted. Seeking treatment for infertility is lawful and legitimate, but there are Islamic objections to some of the modern technologies as reviewed by Hathout (1986).[1] Artificial insemination is to be done with husband's semen and not a donor's, since it is only within the marriage contract that the progeny should be conceived.

In vitro fertilization and similar technologies are permitted only between husband and wife, without the intervention of a third party (alien to the marriage contract), be it a sperm, an ovum, an embryo, or a uterus. The permissibility applies only as long as the marriage is valid, but if the union is dissolved by divorce or death, the mating is no longer lawful.

Surrogacy is outright unacceptable, but in a dispute between the woman who donated the ovum and the woman who carried and gave birth to the baby, the ruling is in favor of the latter. To overcome the problem of surplus of fertilized ova denied the opportunity of later replacement into their mother's uterus, it is recommended that only the number of ova which will be replaced into the uterus be fertilized. Only unfertilized ova are to be kept in cold storage, to be drawn from until the desired pregnancy is achieved. The prescribed limitations would result in a greater cost and the expenditure of more time, but these are of less importance than respect for human life.

Neogenetics has opened new fronts and posed many questions calling for juridical answers. Whereas no ban should be put on scientific research for the sake of furthering knowledge and revealing God's traditions in His creation, "the admission of the fruits of research into the realm of application should be based on careful scrutiny and filtering through the sieve of the *Shari'a*. Genetic engineering to provide adequate supplies of therapeutic drugs is commendable. Prevention or cure of genetic disease by gene replacement is merely a transplant surgery at the molecular level and is permitted. Recombinant DNA technology is obviously wrong when exploited in the field of biological warfare.

Gray areas exist, however, and considering the possible identification of behavioral genes, we can ask what will happen if science slides from the goal of curing illness to that of improving human stock? And who decides what comprises improvement? And, with the potential of blurring the genetic identity of species--including the human species by exchanging sizeable cuts of genetic material, would the scientist be tempted to push on with the experiment in order to assuage scientific curiosity?

It seems that, with the green lights a lot of red lights should have their place along the path. Atomic fission has given us two lessons: that not all harm to come can be anticipated, and that not all harm done can be retrieved. However, the stakes in neogenetics are much greater. With the advent of the Human Genome Project several reservations were rightly expressed, and it seems that they can be suitably addressed under a new order different from our present one.

The division of people into categories classifying them as normal and abnormal will be shattered; the majority of us will belong in a vast gray area as it becomes possible to read individual genomes. A new social order should see to it that no one experiences discrimination on account of his or her genes. Foreknowledge of disease or predisposition thereto can be put to good use in counseling for marriage and career planning as well as for taking protective measures against illnesses. A person genetically predisposed to alcoholism may therefore refrain from drinking and fare better than a "normal" person who allows himself or herself to drift into addiction. Obsession with physical abnormality as a reason for explaining behavioral aberration should be curbed, since the majority of crime and human tragedy is brought about by very normal individuals.

With neogenetics, miracle cures will be available. But these will be quite expensive due to the high expectations of those who have invested an enormous amount of capital into their research and development. A crisis of accessibility and equity will be inevitable unless the system changes to a more "Godly" one. The function of capital and its social obligations should be rewritten, for the bankruptcy of the communist system is no attestation to the health of contemporary capitalism. Social cohesion should curb the current emphasis on individualism under the prevailing pleasure-seeking ideology. When one counts the dollars given away in lotteries and sweepstakes, added to those consumed by drugs, alcohol, smoking, prostitution, and pornography, and those spent in combating them or treating their health complications, let alone money spent in producing destructive arms for stocking, use, or sale, one can't help feeling that the money is there but the priorities are mixed up. This has to change, not only by law--for the law cannot be effective in a moral vacuum--but by changing people and re-educating man who has reached the moon, to reach the heart of his fellow man. The primary ownership of the creation belongs to the Creator, and the mandate delegating it to Man stipulates that mankind should manage it upon the rules of the Owner.

CONCLUDING REMARKS

Developments in biomedical science and technology are occurring at a rapid pace and further acceleration is expected in the future. Lest progress become like a ship without a rudder, ethical guidelines should keep pace with fresh events. The commonalities between the three monotheistic Abrahamic religions are so great that the prospect of a Judeo-Christian-Islamic ethics is not unfeasible. Even if full concordance does not occur, it would be beneficial for our respective communities to identify the areas of disagreement. To discover that we have more in common than we are aware of is certainly conducive to goodwill based on mutual understanding. And where we disagree, we should respect our differences, each following the line that reflects his or her convictions. Resorting to our religions to formulate our ethics is only consistent with our faith in God, and our conviction that this offers us a constant yardstick which is not as subject as other systems to utilitarian perversion or deceitful rationalization. We would like to conclude by an appeal that all will work towards this Judeo-Christian-Islamic code of biomedical ethics.

NOTES

1   Hathout H. *Islamic Perspectives in Obstetrics & Gynecology*, 1st ed., Kuwait: IOMS,1986.
2   Islamic Organization of Medical Sciences. *Human Life: Its Inception and Its End*. 1st ed., Kuwait: IOMS, 1989.
3   International Organization of Islamic Medicine. *Islamic Code of Medical Ethics--Kuwait Document*, 1st ed., Kuwait: IOMS, 1981.

7

A View from Sinai: A Jewish Perspective on Biomedical Ethics

Shimon Glick

It is a formidable and humbling assignment to attempt to represent *the* Jewish dimension of medical ethics in contrast with so many cultures representing billions of humans and millennia of tradition. The task is even more difficult because of the diversity of opinions and approaches *within* the Jewish community. Self-deprecating East-European Jewish humor has often asserted that where there are two Jews, there are three opinions. Israeli governments have fallen over the difficulty in defining who is a Jew. Even David Ben Gurion's poll of dozens of Jewish scholars throughout the world, in an attempt to benefit from their insights on this controversial question, did not settle the issue decisively.

Traditionally, for most of recorded history, one of the singular features of Judaism is its unique amalgam of religion and nationhood. This tight linkage, unbroken for millennia, was disrupted by two movements following the period of the Enlightenment in Western Europe, when the concept of classic religious tradition collided with the wave of intellectual freedom and modernity that followed the French Revolution.

On the one hand, the Reform Jews in Germany denied Jewish nationhood, insisting that they were loyal German citizens of Hebraic persuasion. Conversely, secular Jews, rebuffed by anti-Semitism in their attempts to assimilate fully into European society, created secular Zionism, which focused almost exclusively on the national aspects of Judaism, downplaying the religious elements of the Jewish tradition. Whereas these two divergent streams have moderated their initially extreme positions, the past centuries' crucible of modernity has produced a pluralism in Judaism that makes it difficult to paint a monochromatic picture. The Western world is most familiar with the Judaism of East-European background, whereas the Jewish dispersion is virtually world-wide; communities of Jews have lived in such diverse places as Yemen, Morocco, and Ethiopia for centuries, often in almost total isolation from their co-religionists in Eastern Europe. Thus, one may ask whether an atheistic Marxist Jew in Moscow, an anti-Zionist hasid in Williamsburg, New York, and a relatively unsophisticated village silversmith in Yemen all hold common values. All identify themselves as Jews and lay claim to a common culture. As for their approaches to medical ethics, however, that is my task to distill.

Jewish tradition dates back thousands of years, antedating the traditional Sinaitic transmission of the Torah to the Jewish people, and representing one of the longest known chains of continuous loyalty to the same texts and sancta. Jewish tradition has interacted with pagan, Roman, Greek, Christian, and secular cultures on four continents. In each society, it has absorbed and learned from, as well as contributed to, its environment. Nevertheless, schisms have occurred.

Various deviant Judaic sects have fallen by the wayside. Some have been the direct antecedents of Christianity and Islam, and these faiths often share with Judaism many common values. Jewish culture, at least through its individual representatives, has also contributed significantly to some of the major intellectual revolutions of the past century in the persons of Marx, Freud, and Einstein. Yet, in spite of the incredible temporal, geographic, and philosophic diversity and heterogeneity in Judaism, I believe one can nevertheless extract a cultural core, an essence which may be labeled Jewish. Probably no individual component is totally unique, but the emphasis, the nuances, and the total package are certainly characteristic, identifiable, and unlike any others.

One of the reasons that the core remains, is that groups and individuals who stray sufficiently from the core and succumb to the surrounding culture tend ultimately to assimilate with and be absorbed imperceptibly into that culture, losing their Jewish identity. But the remaining loyal in-group passes the baton from generation to generation with some degree of fidelity.

Judaism is optimistic in nature, having risen repeatedly phoenix-like from the ruins of Jerusalem and the crematoria of Auschwitz. Traditionally, it views the world as being in motion towards eventual perfection and redemption. Ultimately, it is hoped that the world will be altered unrecognizably and will be a fitting environment for the human being, whose own goal is to function in the image of G-d, in the divine model. In the messianic age, human dignity, peace, and social justice will reign, and even life itself will have reached its ultimate perfection--immortality: death will be banned. This vision of a world aspiring to redemption is second to monotheism as, perhaps, a signal contribution of the Jewish tradition to the world. In its broader utopian concept, it has been adopted not only by other faiths, but in many ways even by atheistic Marxism, which fundamentally posits the ability to continuously improve society. In keeping with the concept of a world changing for the better, one of this century's most influential Jewish thinkers, Rabbi Abraham Isaac Kook, regarded Darwin's theory of evolution not as a contradiction to religion, but as a profound affirmation of a paradigm which matched his optimistic view of a world progressing stepwise to a loftier physical and spiritual state.

The Jewish role in this process is the bearing of the responsibility, both as individuals and as a people, for self-betterment and for improvement of one's society in order to eliminate strife, suffering, injustice, and, ultimately in the classic messianic vision, even death. In placing this awesome task upon the shoulders of man, Judaism recognizes his finitude and limitations, but it grants him the inherent potential for redemption by his own powers--if he but acts in accord with G-d's will. This faith in man places upon him the ultimate responsibility for his own actions and their consequences. By following the Divine imperative (the Torah), man can elevate himself above the angels.

The dialectic which expresses beautifully man's appropriate self-image is the prescription by a hasidic sage who suggested that everyone keep two slips of paper, each in a different pocket. On one slip should be inscribed: I am dust and ashes (Genesis 18:27) and on the other: Thou hast made him but a little lower than G-d (Psalms 8:6). One of the slips is to be glanced at when man feels haughty and full of self-importance and the other when he verges on self-deprecation and despair.

The sense of constant striving for improvement, for redemption, which may characterize the Jewish input into diverse societies frequently expresses itself as a source of dissatisfaction and ferment for societal improvement in the spirit of the phrase from the Jewish prayer book, "to perfect the world according to the kingdom of G-d." The Jewish tradition calls upon man not to accept the world as a given, to reject the *status quo* and to ever strive for the triumph of life over death, good over evil, and justice over inequity.

Steeled by adversity, strengthened by belief in G-d and in G-d's ultimate goodness and justice, the Jewish culture has been characterized by an extraordinary ability to cling to hope even in the face of overwhelmingly unfavorable odds. It has shown remarkable survival abilities throughout the centuries in spite of repeated persecution.

In the struggle for survival and the fight for life itself, Judaism assigns to individual human life an intrinsic value, probably higher than any of its cognate faiths. This is perhaps best expressed by the passage in the Talmud (Sanhedrin 37a) describing the creation of Adam: "Therefore was man created as a single human being, to teach that if any person causes a single life to perish, Scripture regards him as if he had caused an entire world to perish, and if any person saves a single life, Scripture regards him as if he had saved an entire world."

This statement highlights the extraordinary value placed on even a single human life, irrespective of its quality, in a totally non-utilitarian way. Life possesses an intrinsic absolute value as a divine gift of creation. In Jewish Halakah (corpus of Jewish law), virtually every religious precept (with the exception of murder, idolatry and forbidden sexual relationships) is suspended in order to enhance even the remote possibility of saving a human life.

Interestingly, even individuals in Judaism who have long abandoned the Orthodox outlook and loyalty, and who may actually be avowedly atheistic or agnostic, still cling to these values. Examples of this behavior can be found in the unusually high dialysis rate seen in Israel which is well beyond what might be expected from Israel's expenditures on health, and far higher than many wealthier countries. The extreme preoccupation with providing care by physicians at the front line of the battlefield is another manifestation of this ethos. Also, in keeping with the higher value placed on human life, there is a remarkable and legendary Jewish affinity for the medical profession in almost all societies, even those where the economic rewards are limited.

Consonant with the high priority given to life, the Jewish tradition, unlike Anglo Saxon law, *requires* the physician to respond to any patient's call for help.[6] This requirement to render assistance to someone in distress is not peculiar to the physician, but obligates any individual to come to the aid of a fellow man. To refuse would fall under the prohibition "Neither shalt thou stand idly by the blood of thy fellow" (Leviticus 19: 16). A physician who does not respond to a sick patient's request is regarded as one who spills blood. The corpus of Jewish law goes further in defining the physician's obligation to respond, imposing it even if there is another physician available, "because one is not cured equally by any physician,"[6] acknowledging the vital role of patient confidence in the particular physician as playing a major role in the curative process.

But, just as the physician is obligated to render care, so too, the seeking of care by the patient is mandatory. The reason for this obligation is that, in our Jewish tradition, man does not possess title to his life or his body. Man is but the steward of the divine possession which he has been privileged to receive. The terms of that stewardship are not of man's choice, but are determined by G-d's commands. We forbid suicide and require man to take all reasonable steps to preserve life and health. When beneficence conflicts with autonomy, the former is given precedence by Judaism, a view clearly in conflict with the modern Western consensus. While such a violation of autonomy for the patient's good is not enforceable in our modern pluralistic societies, it has full sanction in the Jewish tradition, and Jewish courts may enforce medical treatment when unequivocally indicated. Even in modern Israel, unlike the situation in most Western countries, the courts have not decided unequivocally for autonomy over beneficence.

In keeping with the high value placed on human life and the treatment imperatives, it is not surprising that active euthanasia has no place in Jewish tradition. Prayer for death to relieve suffering is mentioned favorably in classic Jewish sources, but never direct action. On the other hand, in the face of terminal illness accompanied by suffering, one is not obliged to prolong the dying process by futile and/or distressing forms of treatment. Indeed, in a moribund patient, traditional sources permit cessation of acts which prevent death.

In their long and often difficult history, Jews have learned to accept suffering as an inevitable concomitant of human destiny on earth. But Judaism finds fewer redeeming features in suffering than do other faiths, and it is fully committed to the use of all the resources at its disposal to mitigate, if not eliminate, suffering to every possible extent. In the terminally ill patient, where there is often a conflict between the control of pain and the desire to prolong life, we permit the treatment of pain even at the risk of shortening life. The delicate line that often must be drawn between hastening death and not prolonging life is difficult and taxes even the most conscientious physician.

The intense respect for human life as an intrinsic value, irrespective of its quality, has for centuries been shared by Christianity and Islam, although perhaps with not as great an intensity. But clearly within the Western world there has occurred an initially subtle, but by now a dramatic and fundamental downgrading, of the value placed on life itself. The recent Hastings Institute publication[2] on the termination of treatment and care of the dying specifically offers four basic principles providing the ethical framework for such decisions, but expressly excludes "sanctity of life" and labels it as a "presumption." Similarly, the Appleton Consensus[5] on guidelines for decisions to forgo medical treatment, while also choosing four basic principles, three of which are identical with those of the Hastings group, also omitted a "respect" for life. The few dissenters from this exclusion, interestingly enough, were those whose loyalty was to Judaism.

In today's society where cost-benefit considerations are increasingly heard, where discrimination against the aged is often supported by politicians, ethicists, and physicians alike, the Jewish tradition finds itself more and more isolated. Similarly, in the controversy about the withdrawal of food and water from the terminally ill or those in the persistent vegetative state, the Jewish tradition rejects the shortening even of a seemingly meaningless life.

While standing in awe of Nature, its wonders, and its Prime Mover, the Jewish tradition does not recoil from interference with "natural law." In the deliberations as to permissibility of a given act, its being "natural" or "unnatural" plays a little role. In our tradition, the world is regarded as a deliberately unfinished product placed in the trust of man--himself a finite and imperfect being. Man is expected, indeed commanded, by an *imitatio dei* imperative to engage in completing, as it were, the work of the Creator. The support for this view is exemplified by the midrashic interpretation of a verse in Genesis describing the Creation whereby G-d "ceased from all His work, which G-d had created to do" (Genesis 2:3). The Midrash relates that the phrase "created to do" means that the world was created with much left "to do." The finishing touches, as it were, are assigned to man. The physical act of circumcision is viewed by some commentators as symbolic of man's assignment to complete G-d's unfinished creation. Man is similarly expected to strive to perfect himself and his society morally and spiritually.

Man is neither to worship Nature as do the pagans, nor is he to be intimidated by it. He is commanded to control Nature and to exploit it constructively. Healing the ill, as but one example of such an endeavor, is therefore not only theologically acceptable, but is mandated. This eagerness to modify Nature, together with the great value placed on human life, contributed to the exalted place occupied by the healing profession in Jewish tradition, transcending the millennia and the diversity of geographic locales throughout the Diaspora. It is no coincidence that so many great rabbinical scholars, particularly in the middle Ages, were also physicians and that the proverbial "Jewish mother" aspires so earnestly to be able to boast of "my son, the doctor."

This strongly positive attitude toward medical intervention, now taken for granted, was not always unanimously held in the Jewish tradition, nor was it itself evident. In the typical Talmudic derivation from a Biblical source, this view is based on the verse dealing with compensation for personal injury: "He must pay for the loss caused by absence from work and cause him to be thoroughly healed" (Exodus 21:19). From this it is derived that *permission* is granted for the physician to heal. The commentators state that the reason that permission is required is so that the physician will not hesitate to respond on theological grounds to the question: How is it that G-d makes one sick and the physician dares to heal? Maimonides, the great medieval Jewish rabbi, philosopher, and physician, and ever the rationalist, expressed this theological justification for medical intervention in a much more pointed fashion in one of his medical treatises.[4] He compares the sick man who declines medications, preferring to rely on prayer, to the man dying of hunger who declines food, choosing instead to await the mercies of G-d to rescue him from the "illness" called starvation.

It is fair to point out that there were trends in the Jewish tradition which looked askance at seeking medical cures for what was perceived as Divine punishment. Yet the mainstream accepted the theological validity of medical treatment and mandated it for both patient and physician.

Judaism respects not only human life, but all life and indeed all of creation, living or not. But there is, in the Jewish tradition, a clear hierarchy in Nature, rising progressively from the inanimate through the plant and animal, to the human and the divine. In a purposeful universe, those in the lower category serve the higher forms. Thus, unlike some modern philosophers who decry the discrimination between man and animal as "speciesism," a concept akin to "racism," our tradition regards such blurring of the boundary between animal and man as more likely to lower man to the level of the animal than the reverse. The use of animals for medical research is regarded as laudable and mandatory when indicated, provided such activity is carried out with sensitivity and a minimalization of animal suffering. But, the license to exploit animals specifically excludes killing and hurting of animals for trivial purposes such as hunting, cockfighting, and the like which have traditionally been totally alien to Jewish culture. Indeed, Albert Einstein is quoted as once defining a Jew as one who derives no pleasure from hunting.

With the Earth and its beauty placed at man's disposal for use and positive exploitation, the Jewish tradition has shied away from asceticism of all kinds, even for its clergy. Failure to enjoy the resources of the universe is regarded with suspicion, almost as a sort of deviant behavior. The ideal human behavior is not withdrawal from the pleasures of life and the manifold gifts of Nature, but the proper and limited exploitation of each and every resource--always with external controls--within moral and ethical limitations, and not in an animal-like fashion.

This delicate balance extends to every area of human life. There is hardly a moment of the day, an area of involvement, or a resource whose use is not regulated by the all encompassing laws of the Torah.

In the area of reproduction, the Jewish nuances are unique. Celibacy, as a form of asceticism, is interdicted. The first commandment of the Bible is: Be fruitful and multiply (Genesis 1:28) and it applies to scholar and ignoramus, saint and sinner. Thus, unlike other faiths where the most talented representatives of society have often committed genetic suicide, the rabbis and scholars usually produced the most progeny. This practice may have had positive eugenic effects on the Jewish population.

Procreation is encouraged, while mutually satisfying sexual relationships within the confines of monogamous heterosexual marriage is not only permitted, but is mandated, even when procreation is not possible because of age, sterility, or other problems. Celibacy as a means of contraception or for any other reason is unacceptable. Man's intervention in the enhancement of fertility, within certain bounds, is encouraged. The integrity of the family unit is a value to be cherished and secured, as is the identity of one's lineage. The profusion of surrogate parenthood permutations and combinations, with potentially far-reaching familial and perhaps societal disruption, is not looked upon favorably.

The enormously high value placed on human life in Judaism does not begin with birth. Potential human life, too, is highly regarded, through technically there is a continuum going back to the sperm and ovum, through the zygote until birth. At no stage is potential human life to be treated casually, but is to be preserved and cherished. Thus, casual contraception for "trivial" reasons and certainly abortion are interdicted. Nevertheless, there is a clear priority given to the life of the mother over that of the fetus, and abortion is permitted, and even mandated, where serious threat to the life of the mother is involved. With the moment of the birth, the infant, normal or deformed, acquires full human rights. Infanticide, now achieving a new rebirth in some respected philosophic circles, is abhorrent and never acceptable.

The Jewish position on homosexuality is unequivocal, regarding it as destructive abnormal behavior. The possibility that homosexual tendencies may indeed reflect an inborn *tendency* does not mitigate the abhorrence that Judaism has toward the *practice*. Just as limitations are placed on heterosexual behavior in spite of the powerful desires that often need to be suppressed, so too does the tradition differentiate with respect to homosexuality between the tendency and the practice.

There is one area of modern medical practice which does not present serious bioethical dilemmas in most of the Western World, but which actually became a major societal controversy for many decades in Israel. The Jewish tradition includes not just a reverence for the human being while alive, but extends a measure of protection to the body even after death. Disrespect for the body, which once was a bearer of the divine soul, is considered highly inappropriate. Proper respect for the body in Jewish tradition requires early burial of the body in an intact state. Indeed, the obligation of burial is so highly regarded that even the Jewish high priest in the time of the Temple--who was not allowed to defile himself by contact with a corpse (even that of his family)--was obliged to participate personally in the burial of an individual who had no relations or friends. Such an act of care and respect for the body of an unknown and unwanted person is regarded as an act of supreme loving kindness, since no recompense of any sort is possible. Thus, in the Jewish tradition, it would be unthinkable to use for anatomical dissection the bodies of the poor unclaimed dead, for these would have the highest priority for respectful burial by the community. This respect for the dead presents a problem in the area of post-mortem dissections, which are permitted by the Halakah only where relatively immediate benefit can be expected to accrue to another person sick with the same illness. The degree of immediacy required for autopsies to be permitted is interpreted variously by different experts, but on the whole, the inclination in the Jewish culture is one of reluctance to consent to autopsy and dissection of the dead.

Where do the traditional Jewish sources stand on medical research, on exploring the universe, on probing its mysteries? Are there limits to the incessant curiosity of the scientist? From the very first chapter of the Bible, man is commanded: Be fruitful and multiply, fill the earth and subjugate it (Genesis 1:28). The phrase "subjugate the earth" has been interpreted by Jewish sages from time immemorial as a mandate for humans to use all physical, mental, and spiritual resources to understand, control, and exploit the environment, presumably in the service of God and humanity. This is a general command to all humankind and not specifically to the Jewish people.

There are at least two further facets to this approach. Maimonides, in his definitive halakic work[3] confronts the difficult philosophic problem of how to fulfill one of the cardinal tenets of the Torah, that of love of G-d: "You shall love the Lord, your G-d" (Deuteronomy 6:5). How can one command or mandate love, which is basically a matter of emotion and which is difficult, if not impossible, to control by command? Maimonides prescribes one method for achieving love of G-d, namely by a study of Nature. "When a man contemplates the world and its creatures, he sees the wisdom of G-d in all that is created and thereby increases his love for G-d. His soul and his flesh thirst for and desire to love the Almighty."[3] In essence, this is understood as a clear religious command to man to explore in depth the wonders of nature--what we would call "pure" research.

Medical research, of course, has additional positive justification beyond that of other scientific research in Jewish tradition, since the preservation of human life has an extraordinarily high priority. Clearly then, research, and certainly biomedical research, is to be encouraged and is looked upon favorably. Historically, medicine was the one secular profession that not only was not questioned by medieval Judaism but was actually taught within the walls of some Jewish institutions of religious learning--since it was not considered a secular study, but a holy calling.

Yet religion in general has classically been associated in the minds of many with restrictions on open and free inquiry, and Judaism too has been tainted with this image. But if one examines classical Jewish sources, one finds encouragement to engage in free inquiry, certainly in the field of science, but also in other scholarly endeavors, with little regard to the consequences of the search. The Talmud has dozens of synonyms for the word "question," and the entire Talmudic process is one of dialectical give and take, of hypothesis, theory, and refutation. In this process, not just the final conclusion is important, but also an understanding of the rejected position, of the alternate possibilities. This, in fact, may be one of the seminal contributions of the Talmud--a spirit of debate, of inquiry, of respect for opposing points of view.

A student is encouraged from early childhood to ask "good" questions, which are defined as those which point out inconsistencies, which shake colleagues out of their complacency, which lead to new insights. New insights, new perspectives are the ultimate goal. Isaac Rabi, the Jewish Nobel Prize winner in physics, is said to have attributed some of his scientific achievements to his mother, who would ask him daily on return from Hebrew school: Did you ask a good question? There are several hundred places in the Talmud where the conclusion is left open--the question persists--no answer is given--and this uncertainty is not considered disturbing.

Rabbi Joseph Soloveichik, one of the great Talmudic scholars of our age, is quoted as telling his students: One does not die from a question. Thus one is not to fear difficult questions, even those with no immediate answer, because these questions, if asked openly and faced honestly, often lead ultimately to solutions and to conceptual breakthroughs, whereas a simplistic, but erroneous, answer may perhaps be the greatest block to progress in Talmudic studies as well as in scientific research. Yet, in the area of medical research, no nation can afford to be more sensitive than the Jewish people to the abuse of research subjects, to making man a means instead of an end. The scars of the Holocaust are still fresh in the minds or our people, and Mengele's survivors still are alive to testify about the degradation to which scientists and physicians can sink in the absence of loyalty to moral and ethical imperatives.

The lessons of the Nazi medical experiments are universal, particularly when one realizes that these horrors arose in what was considered perhaps the most technologically advanced and highly cultured Western country. Alexander, a psychiatrist at the Nuremberg trials, best explained the genesis of the physicians' behavior in a classic article[1] written after extensive research and interviews with the war criminals. His conclusion was that the degradation of German medicine was part of a gradual abandonment of the Judeo-Christian emphasis on the intrinsic worth of each individual and its replacement by a utilitarian ethic. He illustrated this development in German elementary school mathematics textbooks which provided questions such as: "How many apartments for young couples can be built with the money it costs to support a mentally retarded person in an institution for a year?" Even at that time, Alexander detected the first traces of similar approaches in the United States. What can we say today?

One of the questions that naturally arises is: To what extent can so ancient a tradition cope with the complexities raised by the biomedicine of the twenty-first century? This challenge seemed much more formidable and telling several decades ago when science and technology appeared to be all-powerful and when religion was retreating throughout the Western world. But, somehow, the overconfidence of scientism has mellowed in the wake of Auschwitz and Hiroshima. The revival of religion after decades of brutal suppression in different parts of the world has forced serious thinkers to regard some of the ancient verities with greater respect. The Jewish halakic tradition, dating back to Sinai, presents an elaborate legal and ethical corpus based on eternal values. It has demonstrated remarkable resourcefulness, vitality, and adaptability in successfully coping with some of the most complicated ethical dilemmas throughout the ages. I am confident that its eternal values will continue to be a source of divinely based ethical guidelines in the exciting years to come.

NOTES

1   Alexander L. Medical science under dictatorship, *New England Journal of Medicine* 241 (1949): 39-47.
2   Guidelines on the Termination of Life-Sustaining Treatment and the Care of the Dying. *Hastings Center Report*, New York: Briarcliff Manor, 1987.
3   Hilkoth Yesodei Hatorah, *Sefer Hamada* 4: 12.
4   Maimondes, *Treatise on Asthma*.
5   Stanley J., ed. *The Appleton Consensus-Suggested International Guidelines for Decisions to Forgo Medical Treatment*. Appleton, Wisconsin: 1989.
6   *Yoreh De'ah*, 336: 1.

8

Humanism and Eugenics

Ivan T. Frolov

Today, many of the problems that were traditionally considered the domain of science fiction have acquired fundamental significance and have advanced to the forefront of scientific inquiry. The emerging ability to change human nature through eugenics is among the advances opening the door to such problems.

Recent breakthroughs in human biology, genetics, and psychology have enabled human beings to better adapt themselves to natural and manmade environments considerably altered by scientific and technological advances, social transformations, and other factors. These developments open new vistas of active transformation by man of his nature to make it suit better the new tasks that have appeared in cognition and practice and, actually, in all spheres of the life of man as a free and harmoniously developed creature.

Would his physical makeup change? What would be the trends of such changes? Would some new forms of human existence emerge, combined with biocybernetic devices. Would the human race enter a new stage in its evolution at which, to a substantial measure, man would be created artificially. Such a creation would be "manufactured," as it were, with the help of genetic engineering and biocybernetics, thereby producing a "superman" with extra-sensory and extra-intellectual properties--a *homo sapientissimus*.

The term "eugenics" (from the Greek *eugens* meaning well-born) was introduced by Francis Galton in *Hereditary Genius. An Inquiry into Its Laws and Consequences* (1869). The book demonstrated that man's heredity, like that of any other living creature, is governed by common laws of genetics. The author also defined the problem of improving human heredity by increasing and selecting useful qualities and reducing or overcoming harmful ones. Since the latter's frequency correlates with the frequency of marriages between close relatives, efforts to limit such marriages through counseling and other measures help to reduce the incidence of harmful forms of heredity. That is the aim of "negative" eugenics which largely coincides with modern medical eugenics. "Positive" eugenics, on the other hand, aims at a broader objective, namely, developing a "new man" through a selection of genotypes among the progeny of persons possessing exceptional mental or physical qualities. That branch of eugenics has been used (sometimes contrary to the intentions of its advocates) by various reactionaries and racists, particularly by the theoreticians and practitioners of fascist "racial hygiene" and genocide.

Naturally, the disrepute that this brought to the ideas of eugenics resulted in its failure, even though in many respects, it relied on genetically well-established hypotheses and the authority of prominent scientists known for their humanistic views (Nikolai Koltsov, Hermann Muller, John Haldane, Julian Huxley, and others). It is true that basic postulate of "classical" eugenics--concerning the possibility of engineered development, through selection of persons with exceptional intellectual abilities--has met with disapproval by modern geneticists and by the scientists who study human beings in their individual and historical development. This has caused many advocates of eugenics to reconsider some of its original dogmas and to look more closely, in particular, at the social factors in human development. Some of the propositions of genetics, however, remain unaffected by any considerations of social factors.

The evolution of eugenic thought in the USSR is of some interest in this regard. Although often distorted, it merits, at least, some consideration. The eugenic movement in Russia, which arose a long time ago, was formally organized in 1920. It took shape when the Russian Eugenic Society was established in Moscow under the chairmanship of Koltsov, who also took an active part in setting up the *Russkii evgenicheskii zhurnal* (*Russian Eugenic Journal*--seven volumes were published). A second center appeared in 1921 in Petrograd when Yuri Filipchenko organized a Bureau on Eugenics which subsequently served as a basis for establishing a branch of the Russian Eugenic Society. The bureau published *Izvestiya byuro po evgenike pri Rossiiskoi Akademii Nauk* (*Bulletin of the Bureau on Eugenics of the Russian Academy of Sciences*). Of particular interest for the present study are the first three issues (1922, 1924, 1925). Finally, still another institution that concerned itself with eugenics was the Medical-Biological Institute (called the Medical-Genetic Institute since 1935) under the leadership of Solomon Levit. This may be viewed as a third center, for its studies of human genetics and medical genetics were component elements of eugenics. Each of these centers was concerned with specific problems. In particular, the team led by Koltsov studied human heredity in pathological as well as normal states. Its original program for the genetic analysis of human psychology continues to be of great interest today.[6] Geneticists led by Filipchenko were primarily concerned with analyzing the genetics of gifted persons through survey questionnaires addressed to scientists, representatives of the arts, and students. It was also concerned with developing a system of eugenic consultations for young persons considering marriage.[3] The program of the third center envisaged further advances in the twins method for in-depth studies of the role of mechanisms of interaction between genetic and environmental (social) factors in human ontogenesis, studies of the genetics of a number of diseases (diabetes, daltonism, hypertension, ulcers), and analyses of progeny from marriages between closely related persons.[8] Foreign anti-fascist geneticists, including John Haldane, L. Hogberg, Muller, and G. Dalberg, also contributed to the work of the institute.

In an overall evaluation of the eugenic movement in the USSR let us note a significant point: all the programs mentioned were concerned mainly with solving strictly scientific problems.[5]

One should admit, however, that, on the whole, the ideas and works of the foremost Soviet geneticists demonstrated a somewhat simplified and contradictory approach. This is especially true of Koltsov's works. A democratic orientation and a responsible attitude toward using the laws of human heredity and mutability to protect and improve the health of future generations are important characteristics of Russian eugenic thought.

Similar views were advocated at about the same time by Hermann Muller, who worked in the USSR for several years and who actively campaigned for eugenic ideas. This prominent scientist, who made a substantial contribution to the development of genetics, announced a "crusade" on behalf of eugenic measures that were destined, in his opinion, to save the human race from a genetic catastrophe. Initially he proposed the introduction of controls over human reproduction and of selection for improving the human gene pool, to be followed by a program of artificial insemination of women using preserved sperm from outstanding men, drawn from specially created sperm banks. This idea was discussed in Muller's book *Out of the Night: A Biologist's View of the Future*.

At the Second International Congress on Human Genetics (1961), he elaborated that idea in describing his conception of embryo selection. He noted, however, that he could not guarantee complete success since the manifestation of human attributes also depends on the social environment and development.[9] Muller stated: "Only the impending revolution in our economic system, will bring us into a position where we can properly judge, from a truly social point of view, what characteristics are most worthy of a man. . . . Thus, it is up to us, if we want eugenics that function, to work for it in the only way now practicable, by first turning our hand to help throw over the incubus of the old, outworn society."[2] As we see, Muller associated the application of eugenic ideas with specific socio-economic changes in capitalist society. But even the purely scientific aspect of these ideas has met with objections from a number of geneticists, including Theodosius Dobzhansky, George Beadle, and Bentley Glass. Still, eugenics has many proponents among modern scientists, some of whom, moreover, have moved beyond theoretical support to practical activities. An American businessman, R. Graham, energetically supported his friend

Muller. He set up a sperm bank and recruited women who were willing to take part in an experiment to create "superpeople." On Graham's part, this was a rather ill-fated attempt to promote the neo-eugenic ideas of Muller who died in 1967.

Today such projects are often associated with applying to man the methods of genetic engineering, cloning, etc. At the same time, even when neo-eugenic ideas are accepted in principle they often find new substantiations and new forms of embodiment. Interesting data and conclusions concerning the danger of the human race's "genetic degradation" and the ensuing need to adopt eugenic measures are cited, for example, in the survey titled *Biology and the Future of Man*.[1] Its authors believe that no matter how complicated the dynamics of a genetic population, entrance into and interference with it is possible. They envisage that great difficulties will be encountered on this road. Though in principle able to improve his own genetic construction, man is still unwilling to employ this possibility. Selection is a cruel process: swift progress can be achieved solely by restricting reproduction to those whose genotypes exhibit the desired traits. The question arises: Who will be the judge? Which genotypical and phenotypical changes might prove to be optimal? Who will shoulder the responsibility of denying the majority of men and women the right to procreate and of assigning this right to a limited elite group? How will society make the choice?

Will society change so that the self-regulation of human evolution becomes a reality as a result of the fact that the majority of people are voluntarily choosing not to continue themselves in their children? This is highly unlikely in the near future. Mankind, however, may survive for a period long enough to think this problem over and to implement such possibilities.

The survey's authors insist that many differences in mental behavior and social properties can be explained by a qualitative difference in non-genetic factors such as health and strength, intellectual development and background, and life conditions in the earliest period of life. It is now time to realize that these extra-genetic factors determine whether an individual can use his or her genetic potentialities to the greatest degree. Acceptance of these other factors will make it possible to broaden our ideas about already existing genotypes. At the same time, more active studies focussing on the already evident capability of making genetic changes and on the more complete knowledge of gene pools and genetic capacities will provide for the possibility of control of human biological structure possible.

It seems that the road toward achieving a fullness of man's vast potentialities lies not so much in a certain unified form of *homo sapiens* as through a skillful use of man's gene pool changeability. Though standardization is possible, the survey's authors totally reject the appalling thought, suggested by some, that groups of people can be specially selected to perform certain tasks. Together, such a mixture would compose a highly efficient but totally depraved society. If and when man shoulders the responsibility of controlling his own genetic future, his choice should be seriously evaluated and affirmed before proceeding. If a man is prepared to supervise his evolution, he should first formulate the values he is going to attain.

This is, therefore, a humanitarian position. Though failing to determine the specific social conditions under which it can be put into practice, it rejects outright all irresponsible ideas of genetic manipulation that are being revived within so-called neo-eugenics. A number of British scientists have also addressed the need for giving greater weight to social conditions in discussing potential projects associated with a reconstruction of human genetics.[11] They even state that it is desirable to prohibit certain types of research in that sphere due to a possibility that the latter may be used to the detriment of the human race. Many consider such knowledge in itself to be so dangerous that its dissemination should be limited. In a civilization in which the individual is sacred, they state, eugenic procedures are unethical. They point out the fact that the population's genetic structure has not improved through eugenic sterilization, a practice which required great effort even in its introduction. The first stumbling block here is that hereditary diseases are mostly recessive and the bearers of defective genes are widespread in the human population. There is little sense in making attempts to weed out the defective genes, since nature itself prevents their reproduction. The second stumbling block is presented by ever new mutations rapidly taking the place of defective genes which have been weeded out.

Galton suggested that by somewhat increasing the pace of genetic changes in man through eugenics, we imitate, in a more humane and efficient way, natural selection. Genetic engineering, however, is not limited to these specific aims. For example, the idea that a large number of children should be obtained from an outstanding person is potentially dangerous: it enables, for instance, a genetically mediocre but politically successful dictator to disseminate his genes. The idea of attempting to pass on the genes of truly outstanding persons can also be hazardous since we have no exact knowledge of the genetic structure of these geniuses. The authors discuss another possible method leading to humanitarian aims and promoting favorable genetic changes. This method, which can be called phenotypic engineering, is based on our knowledge of blood genetics and includes genetic consultations. All ethical problems in this context hinge on the parents' obligation to take into account genetic information.

British scientists also discuss the problem of whether eugenics is ethically justifiable. They give an affirmative answer to this question since, they argue, as soon as a genetic disease disseminates widely enough, its genetic risk diminishes. For instance, the loss of body hair by our ancestors can be seen as a disease compensated for with clothes designed to save mankind from dying of cold. This example indicated that the current human genetic makeup can be sufficient under certain circumstances and insufficient under others. No exact knowledge of the demands of future civilizations is possible. It would be logical to assume that genetic engineering strives to create a human race well suited to the environment. If this were so, it might be possible to create, in the future, people well suited to live on the moon or in other parts of the universe. But, so far, we cannot forecast the demands of the future.

The advocates of the most recent trends in eugenics, including Elof Carlson, Bernard Davis, Joshua Lederberg, and others,[7] seek to apply the latest advances in modern genetics to restructure man's genotype.

To a substantial extent, neo-eugenics, like eugenic projects in general, seeks to find scientific and personal-emotional support in the idea of an "all-absorbing" concern for man and the human race, for his dignity and freedom, and for his future. In this context, it is assumed that a person who has been subjected to eugenic measures (those of "positive" eugenics) will correspond more closely to his essence. In terms of Muller's classification, such a person would possess strong physical health and mental powers, and greater creativity. Morally, he would be warmer and more sincere in his sympathy for others, would have collectivist inclinations, and would have perceptions which yield a richer understanding of reality and find better forms of expression.

Characteristically, compared to old eugenics, neo-eugenics places a greater emphasis on the means to be used in implementing its projects, on their morality, and on their moral admissibility. Generally, what is proposed is "a noble human form of eugenism" (P. Teilhard de Chardin) which must be applied gradually in the course of centuries, and on a voluntary basis. Moreover, the positions of extreme scientism and socio-biologism, defended by a number of modern neo-eugenists, are being subjected to fundamental criticism "from within," as it were. Obviously, this criticism, motivated by considerations of humanism and an awareness of the social responsibility of scientists, plays an extremely important role in opposing neo-eugenics and is characteristic of many scientists today.[4]

In short, among Western scientists as well as advocates of neo-eugenics and of other approaches that allegedly open the way to a new "fabricated superman," there are many who are guided by a realistic and serious approach to reality and who propose to consider not only the available scientific and technological possibilities, but also the no-less-important socio-ethical aspects of the problem. True, certain advocates of eugenics seek to apply the methodology of a "balanced" socio-biologism that would combine eugenic projects for creating the "ideal man" with social ones. This was clearly seen in the works of Koltsov, Serebrovsky, and also Muller, who believed that programs of planned eugenics would provide the opportunity to make "unlimited progress in the genetic constitution of man, to match and reinforce his cultural progress and, reciprocally, to be reinforced by it, in a perhaps neverending succession."[10] In some respects Muller's position in this regard is close to that of a number of scientists who continue to advocate the idea of creating a "socialist eugenics."

I think, however, that the ideas of neo-eugenics, even in an "ennobled" form, cannot be accepted. These ideas have compromised themselves in the past. Marxist-Leninist theory concerning man and the ways of his development, needs no such "additions," for it already incorporates the findings of science, including genetics, made in the study of man.

Neo-eugenic projects for creating the "ideal man" are unsound, above all, in terms of scientific theory, for they rest on a knowledge of human genetics that is still extremely limited. Further, they are based on false conceptions which link man's genetic foundations directly to his mental and, more generally, spiritual qualities. These projects are fallacious from a social standpoint, for they rely exclusively on genetic factors, rather than on social ones, as regards changing man. Not surprisingly, they have been adopted by advocates of racist ideologies, who promote the theory and practice of genocide. Neo-eugenic projects are also misleading in terms of their philosophical worldview and methodological aspects, for they present a distorted view of man's essence and of his role in the world and in history. They also stand to be condemned from a humanistic point of view because they infringe upon the inviolability and uniqueness of the human personality by promoting scientistic and manipulative approaches to the latter. And finally, neo-eugenic projects should be rejected for moral and ethical reasons, as their implementation threatens the human race and raises doubts concerning such basic values of human existence as love and parental sentiments.

This does not mean, of course, that any intervention into man's heredity is impracticable and undesirable as a matter of principle, and that there will never be any real prospect of changing man's biological nature in a desired direction-- even in the distant future. One must, however, distinguish between scientific feasibility and actual practice. The latter cannot be guided by abstract presumptions and requires a concrete definition of the social conditions which must be met if particular ideas are to be applied. At present, neo-eugenic projects can objectively play and are, in fact, playing a reactionary social role. I am deeply convinced that their application would produce a genetic catastrophe for the human race that would be far more dangerous than the one from which eugenics promises to save us.

While rejecting neo-eugenics for purely scientific as well as social, philosophical, humanistic, and ethical reasons, we cannot ignore the real prospects for man's biological development which are emerging from the research in human genetics that has developed intensively in recent years, particularly in the field of genetic engineering. That research, which has nothing in common with neo-eugenics, reveals new and occasionally equally complex problems. It is, therefore, evident how important it is to discern the social aspects of genetic-anthropological research and their humanistic orientation, an approach which precludes scientistic and manipulative approaches to man and is based on respect for man's freedom and uniqueness.

NOTES

1   *Biology and the Future of Man*, New York, London, Toronto, 1970. For more details see: Frolov I.T. *Advance of Science and the Future of Man* (in Russian) Moscow, 1975.

2   Golding M.P. Ethical issues in biological engineering, *Ethical Issues in Modern Medicine*, 72.

3   Filipchenko Y.A. *What is Eugenics?* (in Russian) Petrograd, 1921. The program of the Bureau of Eugenics is presented in this popular pamphlet.

4   Frolov I.T. *The Prospects for Man* (in Russian). Moscow, 1979, 238-240.

5   Frolov I.T. and Pastusny, S. *Die Evolution des russischen Eugenik--Kritik der Neueugenik--Eugenik*. Jena:Entatehung and gesellschaftliche Bedingtheit, 1984.

6   Koltsov N.K. A genetic analysis of man's psychological features, *Russkii evgenicheskii zhurnal* 1923;1:3-4.

7   Kerimova A.D. Social-ethical problems of human genetics, *Voprosy filosofii,* 1980;5.

8   Levit S.G. Genetics and pathology and the modern crisis in medicine. *Medico-Biological Journal* 1929;5. See also in the same issue: Serebrovsky, AS. Anthropo-genetics and eugenics in a socialist society. The substance of the program was contained in these articles.

9   Muller G. Means and aims in human genetics, *Ethical Issues in Modern Medicine*, California, 1977;60-64.

10   Muller G. *Studies in Genetics*, New York, 1962, 500.

11   *The Social Impact of Modern Biology*. London, 1970.

9

From Medical Deontology to Bioethics: The Problem of Social Consensus of Basic Ethical Issues Within Western Culture and Beyond It in the Human Family

Enrico Chiavacci

MEDICINE

Point One

The main issue in medical ethics has been, and perhaps still is, loyalty to an implicit agreement between doctor and patient.[19] The patient is to be assured that: (a) in any situation the doctor will avoid harming him or her (*primum non nocere*); (b) to the best of his or her ability, the doctor will cure the illness. This kind of medical ethics is, perhaps, better defined as "medical deontology": it is something which rules the behavior of every medical professional, whatever his or her own philosophical or religious tenets might be. It is a type of socially recognized contract which also affects relations between medical professionals: but this side-issue is of no direct consequence for our theme. The ethical viewpoints of doctor and patient will, of course, limit, in some extreme conditions, the respective options. It is something which might occur, but it is not the main issue of traditional medical ethics.

Medical science and practice is today confronted with new tasks. Technical facilities allow doctors to intervene in almost all fields of human life and behavior. Not only can medicine offer treatment for an illness, but it can also offer a better quality of life. It can enhance physical strength or mental capacities; it can help one to sleep or to remain awake; it can prolong life; it can help one to live when any real therapeutic treatment is useless. The combination of medicine and psychology enlarges the scope of medicine from merely restoring physical fitness to that of restoring psycho-physical well-being. I will go deeper into this in Point Three, but it is already clear that we need a better description of what medical ethics should be.

Point Two

When there is an ethical dilemma, I begin by assuming the following:

- There is a choice between different possible options for behavior.
- There is a choice based ultimately on some basic premises; such premises consist of values or principles which are not consequences of other major values, but instead are accepted for themselves.
- There is a choice which, in some way, is a concrete expression of the supreme sense of one's existence.

In the tradition of medical ethics, loyalty to the patient is an ethical choice insofar as it is derived from love or respect for another human being; but the choice can also be derived from the social necessity to respect the implicit agreement, an act that permits serenity and satisfaction. Such a choice may also be one of the basic premises according to which one lives life. Whatever the premise, the ethical basis for the doctor's choice depends on the relation between two single individuals. This ethical basis can be limited in two ways. There are limits imposed by the loyalty of the doctor to the medical profession: these limits are usually implicit in the doctor-patient covenant. There can also be some limits posed by the basic ethical premises of the doctor or the patient. The doctor and patient may have ethical standards which might affect the simple pact as described in Point One.

The patient may ask for an abortion or for treatment for certain sexual dysfunctions, and these requests may be for therapeutic purposes. But the doctor may refuse them on moral principles, although he or she may not impose a personal moral code on patients. There must be an honest explanation of the possibility and the effectiveness of such procedures and a referral of the patient to other colleagues.[13] On the other hand, the doctor may be the one to suggest such procedures: the patient may know their effectiveness, but refuse them on moral principles.

So far we have defined traditional medical ethics as an implicit, basic, socially approved agreement, with some limits in particular cases.

Point Three

Today's medicine does not offer only a specific treatment for a particular illness or pathological condition. It also offers treatments for other purposes. In a more general way, the goal of medicine can be described as intending to *improve the quality of life of human beings, inasmuch as it depends on physical and psycho-physical conditions*. This general description of medicine requires traditional medical ethics to adapt in many ways.

In this emerging role, the traditional therapeutic function of medicine is included, but only as *one* of the areas in which it is involved. As a result, recurrent ethical problems are to be studied from a new and more global perspective. Economics, research, and development are all parts of the functioning global network. They affect the availability of kinds of goods, even the goods offered by medicine--whether these are offers of medications or of services. At the same time, the notion of human rights, more and more conceived as being derived from the inherent dignity of every human being,[21] requires that the "good" of basic treatments be available to every human, everywhere in the world. As a result of this wider notion of obligation, a problem arises with regard to the balance between spending resources for research which uses highly specialized new procedures, and making available basic kinds of treatment for every individual and every nation on this earth.

Thus, the widely accepted notion of the ethical responsibility of *one* doctor toward *one* patient should be studied in a framework of greater global responsibility in which doctors, researchers, and institutions, would consider:

1. Basic medical needs not yet satisfied for a large majority of today's human family;
2. General needs and development of the human family of the future.

This is to say that there should be distributive justice also in the medical field.

Point Four

Tasks other than treatment *stricto sensu* are incumbent today on the medical profession. To plan a rational program for the general well-being of a group, particularly one with a specific purpose such as sports, working, or space-travel; to research and make available methods for birth control; to research methods for a more satisfactory sex life; to research and make available assisted procreation for non-therapeutical purposes; to study and do research on the possibilities for genetic engineering; to study environmental changes and their impact on individuals or groups, and to engage in preventive medicine: all this is *not to cure, but to take care of* the well-being of human beings as individuals or groups that are part of the whole human family, for today and for the predictable future.

In this way and for these reasons medical ethics must become, and is becoming, bioethics: this transformation is a process all of us are experiencing daily; it is also the process which justifies, and gives sense to, this symposium: it is a process which reveals to us our responsibility for the quality of life of humanity. The present transformation of medicine can bring about this improvement only if properly directed. We need a proper direction of this as it seeks to implement a better quality of life. But what does a better quality of life mean?

The answer to this question depends on the significance of human life and on the connection of human life to the global life of our ecosystem. And this depends, in turn, on the notion of nature and of human nature. A good life, the meaning of human life, the meaning of nature--all are conceived in different ways by different cultures. They can be called, in the mathematical sense of the word, "cultural functions." *There is no single, absolute answer* to these questions of meaning.

Philosophical and religious traditions of each cultural area are dominant factors in the understanding of these three cultural functions: the good life, human life, nature. All of them are related to the ultimate meaning of life. Because of its relation to ultimate meaning, today's medicine cannot be regulated only by implicit or explicit agreements between patient and doctor. Bioethics needs some substantial ethical premises, shared by different groups living in the same cultural area, and by peoples living in different cultural areas.

NATURE

Point Five

In the Western (European and North American) tradition, the dominant ethical premise has been, and still is, respect for nature together with respect for human life. Although it is not possible to discuss the problem of natural law in this paper, it should be remembered that natural law, albeit in different interpretations, still dominates the field of bioethics. Early Christianity derived the general idea of nature and of a nature created by God from Aristotle and the Stoa, as well as from biblical sources. Therefore the structures and the regularities (the internal law and the "entelechia") which are present in nature represent the will of God the Creator. In this way, structures and regularities in the cosmos--in the universe created by God, including the human body--can and must give a serious foundation for an ethical natural law: one cannot violate the rules given by God to his creatures.

This has been, and still is, an important criterion for evaluation in bioethics. As a criterion, it is true for many atheists and agnostics, as well as Christians: their illuministic faith in an absolute Reason and the ability of reason to study and understand natural structures and regularities offers to the agnostic or to the atheist the kind of absoluteness which, to the believer, derives from the will of God. But recently some difficulties have been shaking this relatively simple foundation of bioethics.[5]

The *first problem* is the knowledge of nature. One can think of nature as an object totally external to the human mind, one which the human mind can know.

This objective knowledge of nature gives, of course, an objective and immutable basis for ethics. But one can dispute this objectivity, for many different valid reasons. If nature is what I can perceive through my senses, then what if the mental organization of the mere data of the senses is conditioned, or altogether produced, by the cultural tradition in which I was born? A different perception and distinction of colors in different cultures and in different ages offers a simple example of cultural conditioning in organizing the data offered by the senses. But there is more to be said.

Only in the era between Galileo and the end of the last century has it been possible to speak of an objective knowledge of nature. Any such scientific knowledge can be considered today, even at its best, only an approximation open to new acquisitions. We can assume that this will be the case without ever achieving the final status of complete knowledge. Two cases are here quoted: the first concerning knowledge in physics, and the second concerning knowledge in biology. Until Einstein, (or better, Mach), the equations of cynematics were considered absolute, a sort of final knowledge. But from Einstein forward, they have been considered valid only for practical purposes within a limited field of variation of speed: they are not *the truth* about movement in nature. Until the end of the last century, sexual activity was considered to be only a biological fact. That the brain played a central role on one side, and the psyche on the other side, were completely ignored in sexual ethics. Sexual activity was thought to be that which is needed for procreation, something animal-like, just a response to a stimulus. The sexual purpose of self-realization and its most important function, that of communication between two persons, was entirely missed. In Catholic ethics these ends were recognized only in 1965 by the Second Vatican Council,[5] and a little later in the encyclical *Humanae Vitae* by Pope Paul VI in 1968. The problem, however, is more complex than that and has opened the discussion among philosophers and scientists. Natural laws in biology and biochemistry seem not to be of a mathematical kind; the questions of the reversibility of time, or of the possibility of order in the chaos, have uncertain answers. The studies of Prigogine and Stengers and of their adversaries are to be seriously considered.[17]

It is an open question whether or not our knowledge of nature will ever be objective, let alone final. Ethical norms, derived from natural law, are to be considered *provisory in their roots*, and therefore open to change. It is difficult to think of specific norms as objective in the sense that they are based on knowledge of specific objects external to our mind; they can be objective only in the sense that they reflect the actual and provisory state of our internal elaboration of external data received through our sensorial perceptions.

The *second problem* is the uniqueness of human nature and of our knowledge of it. It is granted that the traditional definition of the human being is *animale rationale*, meaning it is natural for humans to set their own goals and to act in a rational way in order to pursue these ends. But in this pursuit, a modification of oneself and one's environment will occur in order to achieve personal and environmental adaption suited to the task. This means that human beings are part of nature (of the universe, or of creation); therefore the capability for voluntary and purposeful manipulation of nature is part of nature (or of the will of God, the Creator). The ethical problem seems *not* to be: Is it permissible to change nature? It seems to be instead: For what aims and within what limits is it permissible, or even, is it obligatory to change nature.[5] Respect for nature (and for God, the Creator) is, then, no longer based on preserving the inviolability of each single element of the cosmos in its structures and regularities; it is expressed in research of the purposes of nature and of the reasonable means by which we may change it.

Nature must be understood as the process occurring within a global system involving the whole cosmos, including the human family and its history. Human beings and the human family as a whole are, at the same time, *subject* and *object* of any manipulation of nature. It is important to observe that we are still speaking of metaphysics: the "physis" is not available for arbitrary disposal; it is available only for enhancing values and aims (the connection of aims to values seems obvious to me). The great struggle about bioethics in the western culture-- theology, philosophy and science--can perhaps be described as a metaphysical struggle. Many warriors would reject even the term metaphysics: metaphysics as *essentia rerum*, or *entelechia intriseca* of natural structures and regularities, *versus* metaphysics as the global meaning of human life and activity in the cosmos (the creation). Within each group there are different schools of thought. In the wide field of Christian theology there is a strong tension between creationism and eschatology (or between deontology and teleology). The proper order of the universe, as described in the first chapter of Genesis, was usually understood as the description of a golden age, given by God and later destroyed by human sin; it was a good order which must be sought by human beings as an ideal in the practice of virtues and ethical life. But it can also be understood as a general goal for collective human history: it is up to the human family to use its ingenuity and activity to discover and pursue the project of God for humanity and for the cosmos.[14] It is this pursuit that Christian theology has rediscovered in our century, the theology of history.[3] In the following points I hope to show that this new attitude has great relevance for our theme today.

A WESTERN APPROACH

Point Six

Let's consider the discussion on bioethics in the Western cultural area. There is no disagreement about the necessity of a social and global approach to the problems of medical science and medical practice. Every therapeutic procedure, every intervention of preventive medicine, every treatment aimed at a better quality of life is *de facto* socially conditioned: it requires social structures and interaction or, at least, social agreement. For instance, effective care of a terminal patient requires all of the following:

- Close co-operation of doctors, nurses, psychologists and families.
- Some ethical rules or protocols accepted by the board of the care facility.
- Allocation of financial resources, always limited, using reasonable criteria of distributive justice.
- A statement of some basic ethical principles and positions which could constitute a general guide for action and, at the same time, offer a means for the medical professional to avoid lawsuits.

This is only one example. Any medical choice needs, and must respond to similar demands, albeit in different ways and degrees. The complexity and social relevance of any medical decision is well-understood and accepted by the great majority of Western bioethicists--more so, however, in Europe than in United States.

The serious problem confronting bioethics is obvious: if a medical decision is dependent on, or relevant to the social life and the good life of a community, then what can be the source of authority for the rules of such a complex system? And who is empowered to determine the criteria on which such rules are based? I think that a social consensus of some kind is required to establish such an authority and such rules. Whatever a doctor is doing for the health or quality of life of his patient can help or endanger or limit care of the health and quality of life of closely related others and, in a more general way, of the whole community and the human family. As for the possibility of a social consensus, I think there are two major difficulties: the first is financial, the second is philosophical.

First Difficulty

We should never forget that medicine is big business. Its activities are for profit, at least in the Western economic system, and include: research and production of drugs and medical instruments; production and distribution of drugs, some of which can lower the quality of life and even endanger it; management of medical institutions and schools; and finally, research and development of biotechnologies. These activities, however necessary, are *not aimed* at improving of the quality of life; they are aimed at the maximization of profit. A few big corporations are in control of the entire market: a shocking survey of the business in biotechnologies was published recently by *The Economist*.[1] Moreover, large corporations make extensive use of advertising, with the medical profession as one target and the common people as another. In this way, the very idea of what people consider to be a good quality of life can be manipulated by the media, according to the financial interest of the corporations operating in this field.

Second Difficulty

Until this century, the great majority of people in the Western cultural context were professing a more or less Christian faith and were obedient to religious authorities. Moreover, the basic idea of nature and of natural laws, which can be valid for believers and non-believers alike, was undisputed, at least for practical purposes: the *etiamsi daremus Deum non esse* of Hugo de Grootes is to be remembered in this regard.[20] But, during the course of our century, this social condition has radically changed. We have already studied the discussion among Christian theologians; but the gnoseological discussion on the ability of human reason to know nature and its laws remains a problem for every thinker, believer or not: there is a crisis of reason. On top of all this, ethnocentrism has come to an end: the studies of social anthropology in the Western culture have demolished the deep-rooted delusion of *being the best*; and rightly so. Together with the new contacts with, and the consequent knowledge of other cultures and cosmologies, this change has opened new insights in Western philosophy and thought. Today's moral theology is also involved in the very difficult process of bringing the ideals and the ethical basis of the Gospel to different cultural patterns.[3]

Point Seven

In Europe, this new condition is known as "pluralism." A social consensus is possible, and easily founded on the notion of democratic *rules of the game*; it seems very difficult, if not impossible, to find a social consensus on the *aims of the social game*; however, it seems very difficult, if not impossible, to find a social consensus on the *aims of the social game*. What does an expression like "a good life" mean? There is no commonly accepted answer to this and to similar questions. "The good life" is a notion which implies a vision of good relations between human beings, and of human being to the cosmos. The first relation, that which occurs between human beings, implies the discussion on human rights, on contractualism, on the welfare state, and so on. The second relation, that of human beings to the cosmos, implies discussion of the possibilities and limits of scientific research. It also implies the discussion--very hot indeed--on anthropocentrism versus cosmocentrism, and on spirituality versus hedonism.

It is important to have a look at the discussion on human rights. Traditional human rights, starting with Locke, were the rights of individual liberty, rights not to be hindered. Since the *Declaration* (1948) and the *Covenants* (1966) of the United Nations Organization, socio-economic rights and rights to be helped, have become more and more important; among them there is also the right to health and to medical care.[21] The traditions of medical ethics have their foundation in the rights of liberty: the right of the patient to freedom in choosing or refusing treatment, doctors, etc. But in bioethics it is the other side of human rights which must prevail: the rights to basic medical treatment and the conditions for a good life. I would say: there are rights of liberty and rights of solidarity: the community must not interfere with the free choice of the individual; but it must also help individuals, in a positive way, in their own development and realization.[22] The first type of rights is dominant in the United States. The second has deeper roots in European tradition: the post-war constitutions of Italy, Federal Germany, and France are a good example of this tradition.

Point Eight

I think that modern, or postmodern, pluralism in philosophical, religious, or practical *Weltanschauungen* can be a serious obstacle to a social consensus on basic principles of bioethics. But I also think that the recognition of both sides of human rights--as described above--can help to define some basic positive moral responsibility of a community towards its members. And this is something more than a consensus on the rules of the democratic game. In this way it is possible to work out a consensus around a common goal; and the common goal could be shared or accepted by individuals with different *Weltanschauungen*.[7] The green movements are usually composed of people who differ in religious or philosophical or practical attitudes, but who are united by a goal, however unclearly perceived. Along the same lines, the committees which prepared the Brandt Report on hunger in the world (1980)[15] and the Brundtland Report on the ecological problem (1988)[16] were composed of people in search of some common "goals for mankind" (E. Laszlo)[12] not of a common philosophy for mankind.

This attitude of Western culture is not yet clearly perceived, but it is already at work. Ethical committees in hospitals, in communities, and even those appointed by governments are growing everywhere in Europe: they are not yet a success, but they are a sign that even in a pluralistic society there is the need and the possibility of social consensus towards common work and common goals.

Mr. Fanfani, then prime minister of Italy, quoted privately in 1963 a conversation he had with Pope John XXIII, when they were travelling together by train to the Sanctuary of Loreto. The Pope, Mr. Fanfani reported, told him: "When I'm travelling and find a man at my side, I don't ask him where he is coming from, but where he is going to." I think that it is a good description of the way in which a pluralistic society can find a common aim, a common ideal of solidarity.

A TRANSCULTURAL APPROACH

The same kind of problem we have just now studied in the Western culture and in its Christian roots presents itself, on a larger scale, when we try to find a consensus for the whole of humanity. The human family is a social body composed of different religious experiences and ethical systems, different cultural patterns and ideals of a good life, and different social and philosophical traditions.

It is true that today the powers of the Western countries (political, economic, and military) are trying to dominate the world. This is something which has to be firmly rejected. Each people and each culture finds its own dignity within its own cultural identity. Moreover, cultural identities, if properly respected and understood, can offer new richness of thought to the whole human family. Therefore each culture and religion, with its ethical perspectives, must be respected and appreciated. Our Western culture *is not the best*: most of the papers and books on bioethics are still strongly ethocentric, and seem incapable of accepting the simple truth that we western people are only one of the components of the complex system which is the human family.

We have to accept this complexity: this means that we have to accept a pluralism in the human family; we have to learn to live with it. Such is the basic condition for living together; but this also constitutes the major difficulty for living together, for cooperating in the search for a common good. We have to face this paradox.

One thing is sure: we will never improve the health and the life of humanity without setting some goals which could be shared and pursued together by different cultural, religious, and political groups. There are at least three problems which involve the future of humanity, and which can be faced only through the cooperation of all of humanity: the problem of nuclear war and the arms race; the problem of hunger in the world; the ecological problem relating to the problem of sustainable development. If we aren't capable of facing these problems together, the survival of humanity is uncertain and degradation of the quality of life is certain. From the point of view of ethical theories and systems, no matter whether theological or philosophical, this type of problem is completely new. No school of ethics and no religion in the history of humanity has been ever confronted with this kind of problem. It is my opinion that we must search for a new approach to ethics, and especially to bioethics. We need some ethical premises according to which some kind of general planetary consensus can be achieved. For this achievement, I think that the following proposition is indicated: to pursue one's own happiness is not the ultimate sense for one's life; each of us has our own share of responsibility for the well-being of every human being and of the whole human family. If happiness means total self-realization, then there is no happiness without a sincere attitude of attentiveness and of self-giving to the others. This has to be clearly understood: the well-being of the human family is not an accidental limit on the search for my own happiness. It is my happiness, my self-realization, or, at least, a necessary condition for it.

We, Christian theologians, must consider that the commandment of love, and not the natural law, is the ultimate regulator of our moral life. This implies that Christian ethics (and, of course, bioethics) cannot be a sort of catalog or directory of forbidden or imposed behavior for every single choice in life. What a totally dedicated life should actually be, cannot be written in detail once and for all in some sacred book. The Gospel is not a treatise for ethical norms: it is the account of the only life wholly lived in the light of the love of God: "Christ . . . by the revelation of the mystery of the Father and his love, fully reveals man to man himself and makes his supreme calling clear."[6] These are the very words of the Second Vatican Council. Thus we have a supreme call[8] and the task of making it concrete through the long process of human history.

The same reconsideration of *ethics as a process*--a process of studying and discovering the best way of realizing the supreme sense of one's existence: in every concrete structural and cultural condition--could, I think, be accepted today by most religious persons and philosophers. *If this is possible*, then the problem of the consensus shifts from fixed religious observance (fundamentalism), or philosophical lack of certitude expressed in endless analysis or skepticism, to the supreme sense of human life. And if a consensus can be achieved, in which the responsibility towards human beings and the human family is essential to the sense of one's existence, then the first step to a transcultural foundation will be paved.

Before us we now have the wide field of concrete choices: incorporating the premises of ethics is now an aim for humanity and every individual; every choice must be measured primarily on the basis of the results of this endeavor. It will be the role of the individual conscience, of religious or cultural institutions, of theologians, philosophers, and scientists, to search for the best way of striving for this goal, with regard to the variety of historical, social, and cultural conditions in which the one target shall be pursued. In this way, the cultural identity of each group is safeguarded. An open and continuous dialogue between the people and scholars living under different conditions is required, this symposium is, perhaps, the first serious attempt at such a dialogue. The dialogue is, I think, a basic moral duty.[9] Actually, it is necessary for avoiding biased reasoning and for acquiring new knowledge and new experience of what, in different cultural areas, might be considered either a danger or an improvement of human life. But the dialogue is possible only when there is a consensus on the final goal.

From what I know, many religious and philosophical schools of thought are moving in this general direction. A recent survey of these movements, by H. Kung [11] and K.J. Kuschel,[10] corroborates my position.

There is, of course, the risk of an ambiguous syncretism in religion, and of a dangerous relativism in ethics. Both risks are real. But the challenge to increase chances of survival for humanity and of a better quality of life for every human being compels us to take these risks. *On the danger of syncretism*, I think that all religions should be brought together, having in mind the final goal, not necessarily the rationale or the tenets of faith which support their striving towards goal. Each religion and each culture can and must preserve its own identity; but each must also consider its identity not as a basis for division between hostile groups (as we saw, for example, in religious wars of the past and are seeing again in the present); instead, each identity must be considered as a contribution to the common goal.

On the danger of relativism, as opposed to objective normative ethics, it is to be observed that the duty of living one's life for the good of the human family is a very objective one. There is no place for permissivism: no single human choice is exempt from this duty. But each single choice, or each particular ethical norm, must be based on objective knowledge of human life in the universe, and on objective needs of human beings and groups. This kind of objectivity is not to be confused with a sort of ethical fixity. To interpret objectivity as fixity in moral norms is a dangerous intellectual move common to every institutional religion.

And it is particularly dangerous in bioethics. Knowledge changes every day; needs and dangers of human beings and the human family also change; to be objective, ethics must take account of these changes. There can be, and there are, in fact, some inviolable limits to human behavior; there are actions which are inconsistent with the values implied in the goal. It should be possible to find a large worldwide consensus on a very limited list of such actions[11] such as, for example, the killing of an innocent persons, the wanton destruction of parts of the cosmos, theft and deceit which destroy the reliability of social life, and the breakdown of family life. But every issue has to be very precisely defined; that is the peculiar task of normative ethics, and a very difficult one. Inviolable limits of the same kind should also be established for the objectives in research. But the great majority of our ethical choices should be open to change as a result of new knowledge and even of changing needs of our brothers and sisters.

It is my opinion that bioethics is now imposing new burdens on general theories of ethics and moral theology. These burdens are also a new horizon. We are today at the very beginning of a road which leads to that horizon. Let us go forward.

NOTES

1   A survey of biotechnologies: the genetic alternative. *The Economist* April 30 1988.
2   Chiavacci E. *Teologia Morale: Morale Generale, Vol I.* Assisi: Cittadella Editrice, 1977.
3   Chiavacci E. *Teologia morale: Complementi di Morale Generale, Vol. II.* Assisi: Cittadella Editrice, 1980.
4   Chiavacci E. La teologia della "Gaudium et spes," In: *Rassegna di Teologia* 2:1385.
5   Chiavacci E. Telematica e biotecnologie: che qualità della vita per il domani. In: *Problemi di Bioetica* September, 1989.
6   Concilium Vaticanum II.: constitutio pastoralis de ecclesia in mundo huius temporis (english transl) In: Abbott, WM, ed. *The Documents of Vatican II*, New York: Guild Press-Associated Press, 1966, 22.
7   Ehrlinghagen K., Fundamentalismus in der offenen Gesellschaft. Stimmen der Zeit 3:1590.
8   Engelhardt H.T. Hartshorne, theology and the nameless God, In: Shelp E.E., ed. *Theology and Bioethics*. Dordrecht Holland: D. Reidel Publishing Co., 1985.
9   Habermas J. *Moralbewubtsein und kommunikatives Handeln*, Frankfurt am Main: Suhrkampt Verlag, 1983.
10   Kuschel K.J. Weltreligionen und Menschenrechte. *Concilium* 2:1990.
11   Kung H. Auf dem Weg zu einem Weltethos der Weltreligionen, *Concilium* 2:1990.
12   Laszlo E. *Goals for Mankind*, New York: The Research Foundation of The

State University of New York, 1977.

13 Masters W.H., Johnson V.E., Kolodny R.C., eds. *Ethical Issues in Sex Therapy and Research* Boston: Little, Brown and Company, 1977.

14 Moltmann J. *Gott in der Schopfung: okologische Schopfungslehre, Munchen*: Kaiser Verlag, 1985.

15 *North-South: A Programme for Survival*, The Independent Commission on International Development Issues, 1980.

16 *Our Common Future*, London: World Commission on Environment and Development, Oxford University Press, 1987.

17 Prigogine I., Stengers I. *La nouvelle alliance. Métamorphose de la science* Paris: Gallimard, 1979.

19 Ramsey P. *The Patient as Person* New York: Yale University Press, 1970.

20 St. Leger J. *The Etiamsi Daremus of Hugo Grotius*, Rome: Pontificia Universitas Gregoriana, 1962.

21 UNO, *Universal Declaration of Human Rights*, Preamble.

22 Whitehouse W.A., A theological perspective, In: Dowrick F.E., ed. *Human Rights Durham*: Saxon House, University of Durham, 1979.

10

Biomedical Ethics in the Developing World: Conflicts and Resolutions

B.O. Osuntokun

INTRODUCTION

Health and Economy in the Developing Countries

Many developing countries, especially in sub-Saharan Africa, have certain common characteristics. Their economies have deteriorated over the last decade, with negative, or only small annual economic growth, huge national debts, and a crippling repayment rate of national debts with several countries having interest charges in excess of their annual foreign exchange earnings.[131] Most of the countries have a low proportion of gross domestic product (GDP) --less than 2 percent, compared with 5 to 12 percent in developed countries-- allocated to health care services, and a high percentage (up to 40 percent in some countries) spent otiosely on weapons and armed forces. A large number of these countries have been devastated by wars (some lasting for the past two decades or longer as in Ethiopia, Angola, and Sudan), drought, and failed agricultural policies. As a result, they have suffered widespread malnutrition and explosive population growth. Paradoxically, some of the countries with the poorest health status, as measured by indicators such as infant mortality rate (IMR), life expectancy (LE), and maternal mortality rate (MMR), spend the highest proportion of GDP on weapons and maintenance of armed forces.[65] Sub-Saharan Africa is said to receive annually, external aid of about US $11 billion but spends US $12 billion annually on weapons.[9] By and large the debt crisis has been the most destabilizing factor in these countries: it has been pointed out that, overall, between 1982 and 1987, the developing countries sent to the developed countries a staggering US $220 billion more than they received--a kind of colonial tribute extracted by the rich nations from the poorest people on earth.[4,5]

In many of the developing countries, in addition to widespread poverty, (which is now affecting not only the peasants, but those who were previously regarded as middle class), and the effects of reduction in government or public spending on social services such as health and education, there is gross inequality in the distribution of wealth. A large majority of the population (sometimes up to 80 percent or more) are very poor indeed and lack adequate access to most of the modern necessities of life--clean water supply, nutrition, education, hygienic housing facilities, and health care services. In some countries, especially in sub-Saharan Africa, the health of the population has actually deteriorated compared with the situation a decade ago. In many of the developing countries, the phenomenon of debt-death link has been observed: the more interest payments on national debts, the lower the average life expectancy of the citizens.[111] Because of poor economies, or because of a lack of motivation, many of these countries do not actively support the utilization or pursuit of health research as a tool for development, and do not have or maintain any research infrastructure--including mechanisms for establishing national health research policy, for management of health research, and for control of ethical issues in health care and health related research. It is against this background that one should view ethical issues in health care and research in the developing countries.

UNIVERSAL LANGUAGE OF BIOETHICS AND APPLICATION

In spite of differences in culture and attitudes of peoples in various countries in the world, all should understand and apply the basic principles of bioethics which uphold human rights. These principles include the following: social justice (fairness, equity, equality in allocation of resources for health care); beneficence (doing things that will benefit patients by sustaining life, treating illness, and relieving pain); nonmaleficence or *primum-non-nocere* (first, do no harm); informed (meaningful) consent, including disclosure (providing adequate and truthful information for competent subjects or those with sufficient decision-making capacity); autonomy (freedom to make one's own choices, to exercise individual rights, and to determine the direction of one's own life; acknowledgment and respect for the right of patients to determine much of their medical care); and the right to privacy (to be protected from unwanted medical treatment).[49,64,77,97,113]

The greatest medical-ethical need in developing countries is justice and equity in the allocation of resources and distribution of health care services. It is fortunate that all countries, developed and developing, who are member states of the World Health Organization (WHO) have accepted that the cornerstone of national health care systems is primary health care. Primary health care is essential health care, universally accessible to all, utilizing acceptable efficient technology, affordable to the community, and offering full participation to the individual and community. There is, of course, a huge gap between rhetoric and reality in the performance of developing countries since the primary health care revolution was launched by WHO in Alma Ata in 1978. In several developing countries, as much as 80 percent of the population currently has no access to modern health care services. Gross inequality in access to and utilization of health care services occurs in a few developed countries, notably the United States of America. In 1988, 37 million persons in the United States (17 percent of the population) were reported to have no health insurance, and 13 percent of adult Americans said that medical care needed by them was not available either because it was too expensive or health coverage was inadequate.[17] It is, of course, salutary that in a pluralistic society such as the United States of America, there appears to be a consensus that all should be able to access adequate health care.[14] In countries such as Canada, the United Kingdom, and the Scandinavian and Eastern European countries, with national health service or equivalent (at least in theory), nearly all have access to health care services. There are, however, gross inequalities in the health of populations in some of these countries such as the United Kingdom.[121]

In the ideal situation, health care or access to facilities that would give an individual a chance for good health should be a right.[109] The minimum required to ensure such a right includes the provision of basic public health measures such as education (including health education), environmental hygiene and a clean water supply, adequate nutrition, and other components of primary health care such as maternal and child care, immunization, adequate treatment of common diseases, and provision of essential drugs.

In any society today, it would be insensitive to argue against the right of all to health care. Even in the pluralistic United States of America, as long ago as 1979, a presidential commission stated that society has an ethical obligation to ensure equitable access to health care for all. The aim of this directive was that a standard for adequate level of health care be developed below which no one ought to fall, but not a ceiling above which no one may rise.[57] More recently, in 1990, Davies and Felder, lamenting the American scene, wrote: "We can no longer hold our peace. We see medicine, our profession, the bravest and gentlest of them all, in grave danger. And in that danger, medicine is shutting the door of its soul on the American people and on itself."[35] Davies and Felder went on to suggest that a presidential blue-ribbon commission be appointed to look closely at the following issues, among others: implementing universal health care coverage with reform of the extant Medicare/Medicaid insurance system; control of medical technology; establishing a national medical ethics commission; instituting national malpractice reform; establishing a national health services research institute; improving health promotion/disease prevention education.[35] These suggestions have nearly universal applications, and developing countries would benefit from these ideas.

In all countries, developed or developing, resources for health care are limited, hence justice and equity in allocation of whatever resources that are available must be influenced by the basic principles of health economics--efficacy, efficiency, positive cost-benefit ratio, and cost-effectiveness. Special consideration should be given to high-risk and vulnerable groups such as children, mothers and pregnant women, the elderly, and the poor in "the inner cities." Health systems research and epidemiology and other health-related research should contribute enormously to ensure judicious utilization of available resources. In many developing countries, because of inadequate epidemiological information, resources are often inappropriately allocated and utilized: it is not uncommon for 95 percent of resources for health care to be expended on 5 percent of the causes of ill health. The health care services covered are often dramatic and focused solely on medical care rather than more effectively directed toward health care, as a whole, of which medical care is only a component. Ideally, health policies should be based upon evidence, not opinion or consensus, on the magnitude of health problems to be solved, on the economic consequences of all options and on the estimates of outcomes.[42]

The ethical thrust in emphasizing primary health care, (integrated, of course, with other levels of health care, social justice, and equity in allocation of resources for health care), recognizes the fundamental importance of providing access to essential health care for all, satisfaction of the needs of the many rather than the demands of the few, and the utilitarian necessity to use the limited available resources where they will yield the greatest good for the greatest number for the longest period.[92] The resources available for health care in developed countries range from US $1 to US $100 per capita per year (compared with US $800 to US $2,500 in the developed countries). It is obvious that, if developing countries are to progress, health care services must be based on maximum efficiency and informed management policies and options.

Variable, but generally unsatisfactory, progress is being made by developing countries in establishing national comprehensive health care services[26] and in ensuring that health care is acknowledged as a social right of all citizens. Some developing countries, such as Mexico, have asserted that access to health care is a constitutional right.

The effectiveness and competency of health care systems is often linked to economic development and standards of living. Most people would now accept or agree that the main determinants of the health of a population are not within the control of the medical system. It is, however, equally true that social and economic development cannot be achieved without good levels of health care. While developing countries should aim at self-reliance, external assistance is often required for economic growth: no country in the world, in any case, is totally independent of others. It is ethically justifiable for the richer developed countries to continue to assist the developing countries especially in building health care systems and the use of health research for development.

As a layman economist, it seems to me that it is correct to emphasize that "developing countries need to be relieved of most of their international debts,"[59] for these debts are jeopardizing the health of communities in these countries. Developing countries, especially in Africa, must emulate countries (such as Mauritius) which have managed to pull themselves out of seemingly terminal decline and to achieve efficient political and social management of available resources. Countries that have suppressed political freedom, with a few exceptions, are less likely than others to be concerned with ensuring that citizens have access to health care as a right. (Of the forty-five nations of black Africa, democracy exists today in only six . . . Namibia, Botswana, Gambia, Senegal, Mauritius, and Zimbabwe.)

To argue that the Western developed countries have given US \$230 billion in aid to the African continent since 1960s, and yet that people in most African countries are worse off today than three decades ago,[130] is to miss the point. Africa's lasting solutions lie more in cessation of senseless civil wars raging in at least ten African countries, reductions in stultifying expenditures on the military, the arrest of capital flight,[9] better management of resources, public accountability, and political emancipation and stability.[59]

The health care professions, led by physicians, have an ethical duty to champion the cause of justice, equity, and equality in allocation of resources for health care, of judicious utilization of the resources, and of making accessible efficient, acceptable health care to all. Lundberg correctly emphasized the point when he wrote: "Organized medicine up to and into the next millennium must be obviously in the public interest and of world-wide scope. It must ensure access to care of acceptable quality for all, practice economic soundness, balance health fairly against all other societal needs, emphasize good communications and most of all require and demonstrate goodwill to all."[78]

ETHICS IN HEALTH-RELATED RESEARCH
IN DEVELOPING COUNTRIES

The principles of ethics in biomedical research involving humans and animals, as documented in roundtable conferences of the Council for International Organization of Medical Sciences (CIOMS--a joint WHO-UNESCO body), [11,12,100] should apply in developing countries as well as in developed countries. The CIOMS documents also embody the Declaration of Helsinki adopted by the 18th World Assembly in Helsinki, Finland, in 1964 and revised by the 29th World Medical Assembly in Tokyo, Japan, in 1975.

The cornerstones of ethics in biomedical research involving human subjects are informed, meaningful consent of the subjects and a proper procedure for obtaining the consent approved by an appropriate and suitable qualified body independent of the investigators. Where it is impossible to obtain informed consent, vicarious consent could be obtained from parents or some legal guardian, as with children or the mentally handicapped or incapacitated. Subjects must retain autonomy and be free to withdraw without incurring any penalty such as restriction of access to appropriate health services or infringement of the doctor-patient relationship. Subjects must not be exposed to any unreasonable risks. Mechanisms for assessment of risk and for accident compensation must be built into the research procedure, as specified in the CIOMS document.[100] Concern for the interests of the subjects must always prevail over the interests of science and society, as specified by the declaration of Helsinki.[100]

There are cultures in which the rule on the exercise of autonomy by a mentally competent adult could be modified. In some parts of Africa, the husband's consent must be obtained before that of his wife. In my own opinion, even in this context the husband's consent should not be a substitute for that of the wife, but should be an additional consent which may not override the wife's refusal.

Some have argued that in certain developing countries it would be valid to obtain vicarious consent by community leaders for research involving entire communities or large segments of them, and that, in certain circumstances, once this has been done, informed consent from individuals would not be necessary. I do not agree with this view. The assertions that, in some central African cultures, the concept of "personhood" differs so fundamentally from the one found in Western culture, that "person" as an individual does not exist in the local language of some Bantus, and that "personhood" is defined by one's tribe, village, or social group,[36] can only be true in some small ethnic groups: it is not true of most parts of black Africa.

In my opinion and that of many others, consent by community leaders could complement informed consent of individuals or facilitate obtaining informed consent of subjects as long as the research procedure involves direct contact with individuals. There are instances, however, when the rights of individuals may be secondary to the rights of the community, such as when incidental infringement of individual liberties is decisively outweighed by the benefit to the community as a whole. Examples include research in, or measures involving, modification of the environment (vector control) and research on public health measures (new prophylactic or immunizing agents), new treatment of water supply, and nutritional supplements to staple foods. In such instances, the ultimate decision to undertake the research would rest with the responsible public health authority.[100] And even then, ". . . all possible means should be used to inform the community of the advantages expected from such research and any possible hazards or inconvenience. If feasible, dissenting individuals should have the option of withholding their participation. Whatever the circumstances, the ethical considerations and safeguards applied to research on individuals must be translated in every possible respect into the community context."[100]

In epidemiological research, it is ethically important, especially in developing countries where health care services may be grossly inadequate, that facilities be provided to deal with acute medical care situations and incidental illnesses. It is also important that, when necessary, appropriate steps be taken by researchers to inform the community of the results of their research. In one country in which yellow fever is endemic, researchers found in 1985, serological evidence of low community immunity and published the result in a respected scientific journal. Nothing else was done by either the researchers or the public health authorities (who were unaware of the results of the research). A year later a virulent epidemic of yellow fever broke out.

For international cooperation and national research needs in developing countries, researchers from developed countries are often involved in research on human beings in developing countries. Such collaborative research is usually sponsored by external agencies including international organizations or nationally based funding agencies such as foundations, research councils, universities, and research-based pharmaceutical companies. Ideally, such projects must involve researchers who are citizens of the developing countries where the research is being done. This is to ensure that some technology transfer or building of local problem-solving capacity is involved.

It is unethical to carry out what has been referred to as "parachute" or "helicopter" research projects in which researchers from developed countries go to developing countries, carry out and complete research projects with little or no involvement of researchers from the developing countries, and then leave. In some instances, results of such research projects have been published even before data was shared with the developing countries in which the work was done. The externally-sponsored research project should be approved by the national or local ethical committee in the country where the research is being done, and also by an appropriate ethical committee of the developed country or home countries of the researchers. It is a correct ethical principle which asserts that externally-sponsored research should serve local or national, rather than external interests.

Not infrequently in the recent past, especially in countries where there was no adequate mechanism for management of research and hence no national or institutional regulations on ethics of research involving human subjects, researchers from developed countries have carried out research without apparently complying with ethical guidelines which would have been appropriate or required in their own country. I believe that there ought to be some minimal universal ethical standards which should apply to research involving human subjects anywhere in the world: those already specified by CIOMS[100] are adequate for this purpose. When developing countries (in which externally-sponsored research is to be carried out), do not have national or institutional regulations, the regulations of the developed countries and their institutions who are sponsoring research projects should apply. Cultural modifications such as the additional consent of the husband or of community leaders should supplement, not substitute for, the accepted ethical norm of informed consent of individual. The minimal ethical standards (e.g., those of CIOMS), should, like scientific standards, be regarded as absolute.

In the ethics of research involving human subjects, as in science--and unlike politics--there should be no compromise. I agree with the view that the force of local custom or law cannot justify abuses of certain fundamental rights and that the right of self-determination on which the doctrine of informed consent is based is one of them.[5] When researchers from developed countries compromise the basic ethical principles in research involving human subjects in developing countries, they invite the justifiable accusation of ethical imperialism[5,13] or of exploitation or dictatorship. No research involving human subjects that could not be done in a developed country should be carried out in a developing country. For example, it has been suggested that because human immunodeficiency virus

(HIV) infection is common in certain parts of Africa, testing of low-cost HIV candidate vaccine should be carried out mainly on that continent.[13,27] This would be unethical. Both the developed and developing countries must make sure such an unethical practice does not occur.

The other side of the coin is seen when clinical trials of drugs are carried out in developed countries and the results are then "extrapolated" to developing countries. This could be unethical. It is now well established that there are variations in pharmacokinetics and pharmacodynamics of drugs and of drug toxicity which are related to diet, lifestyle, racially and genetically determined metabolic differences, and genetic polymorphisms. An example of the last is glucose-6-phosphatedehydrogenase deficiency, which increases the susceptibility of black Africans to massive hemolysis in reaction to drugs such as the 4-amino quinolines (primaquine and pamaquine used for radical cure of malaria). The Chinese, black Africans, and Afro-Americans and Caucasians differ in the pharmacokinetics and pharmacodynamics of beta-blockers. The Chinese show a much larger reduction in heart rate and blood pressure and also metabolize propranolol more efficiently than American whites.[135] The reduction of blood pressure by propranolol is less in black Americans than in white subjects.[39] The differences could be partially explained by the variation in the genetically variable member of the cytochrome P450 system known as debrisoquine hydroxylase.[114]

It is well recognized that there are racial differences in other drug-metabolizing enzymes in humans, such as alcohol dehydrogenase and the acetylating enzyme for isonicotinic acid anhydride. Ideally, the multinational drug companies should carry out separate clinical trials of new drugs in major countries and major racial groups. Such differential testing would place unending and unnecessary burdens on both suppliers and consumers of drugs and, hence, it has been suggested that an international organization such as WHO should provide guiding principles.[66] However, it is crystal clear that, based on the evidence available, there is an ethical obligation to assess drug efficacy and effectiveness in different populations in order to detect differences in racial and ethnic groups and to take into account the fact that the results of studies performed on one population are not necessarily applicable to other populations. It is no longer invalid to confine well-controlled studies of drugs, performed before marketing a drug, to groups of patients in Western countries.

A basic principle in therapeutic trials that is related to the issue of racial and ethnic differences in drug efficacy and effectiveness is the concept of exclusion criteria. It is debatable whether it is ethically justifiable to exclude certain patients (on the basis of age, severity of disease, co-existing disease, difficulty in enrolling) from controlled trials in order to obtain "homogeneous groups," and then, after the trials, to extrapolate the results to all groups, including those groups which were excluded from the trials.[25,58]

It has also been suggested that, just as informed consent is necessary for a subject to be enrolled in a research project such as a controlled drug trial, a similar informed consent should be obtained before a subject is excluded from a therapeutic trial which may be potentially beneficial to the subject.[25] "Parallel tracks" are now being created from patients outside of drug trials. These are a result of unwillingness to agree to be randomized or to restriction from the protocol when it is unknown whether the drug will be more helpful than harmful. These "parallel tracks" enable such patients to receive unapproved drugs. This is unethical. What is being suggested is that all available patients who might benefit should be included in a randomized trial.

When research and controlled trials carried out in developing countries have proved efficacious and effective, it is ethically desirable that the new treatment shown to be of value should remain available and affordable to all. It is understandable that market forces are involved in pricing new drugs. An ideal situation is that typified by the availability of *Ivermectin* for mass treatment of filariasis, although special considerations made it possible for the manufacturer to make the drugs available free-of-cost. The opposite situation is the high prohibitive cost of *eflornithine* (dimethylfluoroornithine), the only new drug in three decades to prove efficacious in the treatment of African trypanosomiasis --but at a cost of more than US $280 per course of treatment.

SOME TOPICAL ISSUES IN BIOMEDICAL ETHICS

Progress in biomedical and physical sciences and technology over the past three decades has brought enormous benefit to health care systems. It has also created ethical problems in certain areas, both in medical practice and research. These include: reproductive health, organ transplantation, screening (including prenatal diagnosis of genetic diseases), mapping and sequencing of the human genome and the possible use and misuse of resultant information, dying with dignity (including euthanasia and critical care medicine), the consequences of increasing longevity of populations, and the use and misuse of technology. Other important topical ethical issues of great concern to the developing countries relate to the pandemic of HIV infection and acquired immunodeficiency syndrome (AIDS), alternative medicine, advertising by health professionals, and promotion of pharmaceutical/industrial products.

Reproductive Health

1. In Vitro Fertilization (IVF), Embryo Transfer (ET), and Related Technologies
Although explosive population growth is currently a characteristic of most of the developing countries and is more of a catastrophic bane rather than a boon, childlessness is regarded as a disaster in most communities in the developing countries. If cost were no problem, infertile women in developing countries would certainly seek the benefit of the newer techniques of IVF and ET and related assisted-reproduction technologies. IVF/ET, of course, has ethical problems, even though it has been used successfully as treatment for infertility caused by endometriosis, ovulation disorders, antisperm antibodies, genital tuberculosis, and male factors.[125] IVF/ET benefits only a small proportion

of infertile women and is justifiable only for those with bilateral tubal occlusions. It is expensive; the cost of each live birth by IVF/ET is estimated at about US $50,000.[30,125] IVF/ET has serious health risks as well. These include the following:

- Threefold increase in the risk of multiple pregnancy, since three or more embryos are transferred to ensure success;
- Four times the population rate of perinatal mortality;
- Twice the population rate of neonatal mortality;
- Complications linked with induction of superovulation by fertility drugs (cysts, coagulation abnormalities leading to thromboembolism, stroke, myocardialinfarction, ovarian cancer);
- Bleeding, infection, and injuries to blood vessels and viscera during the retrieval of oocytes; infection during ET;
- High frequency of pregnancy-induced hypertension and high Cesaerean birth rate (over 50 percent).

Quite often, pregnancy reduction is indicated following IVF/ET. This involves locating the fetuses with ultrasound and destroying *in utero* the most accessible, e.g., by injection of potassium chloride into the chest, a procedure considered by some to be an unethical and indefensible act, as abhorrent as illegal killing. Since the first IVF/ET baby was born in 1978, more than 5,000 have been delivered, but no proper evaluation has been carried out with regard to the efficacy, safety, and cost-effectiveness of this method compared with more established treatments for specific classes of infertility. Little is known about the disability rates of children born after IVF/ET, as there are no follow-up studies.[125] Other ethico-legal, social, and religious dilemmas associated with IVF/ET and related technologies include the issues of surrogate motherhood, dubbed "womb for sale," in which women carry embryos for infertile couples; the storage, ownership, and disposal of extra ova, sperm, and embryos; and artificial insemination with sperm from a man other than a woman's husband.[23,79]

Many wealthy, childless women from developing countries have sought the services of IVF/ET clinics in developed countries and will continue to do so. However, on the basis of priorities, needs, and utility calculations, the promotion and development of IVF/ET technology in developing countries is probably unjustifiable. However I know at least one very populous country in sub-Saharan Africa which, following the duping of women by quacks who claimed to practice IVF/ET, has recently begun a serious investigation of the possibility of providing IVF/ET technology. In general, however, developing countries should concentrate on prevention and primary care management of infertility: hence, most financial and manpower resources should be directed toward strategies to prevent infertility through prevention and treatment of sexually transmitted diseases and development and use of safe contraceptive options.[125]

2. Abortion

Important problems in many developing countries include:

- Whether family planning programs should offer abortion services due to the fact that they are often fervently desired by many women under certain circumstances;
- What happens to these women when such services are not offered by family planning clinics.[23]

In a developed country, such as the United States, abortion is said to be, perhaps, the most difficult and most divisive ethico-legal issue facing the country: the latest decision of the U.S. Supreme Court in July 1989, in *Webster v. Reproduction Health Services*, confirmed by a narrow majority the general parameters of an earlier decision in *Roe v. Wade* that the constitutional right of privacy protects a woman's decision as to whether or not to terminate a pregnancy.[7] Abortion is still illegal in a few developed countries, such as Ireland. In April 1990, the King of Belgium, who was childless, abdicated for twenty-four hours because of personal views--moral and religious convictions that abortion is abhorrent--rather than sign a bill legalizing it.[69] In most developing countries abortion is legally permitted to save the life or the health of the pregnant woman, but in a few such countries it is prohibited. However, in most of the countries which have anti-abortion laws, they are not enforced.

The hierarchy of the Roman Catholic Church has been the most vigorous and articulate opponent of abortion, but many Protestant denominations, orthodox Jewish teaching, and Islam also favor anti-abortion policies. The fundamental ethical and religious basis for opposition to abortion is the point at which a fetus/embryo becomes a person--at fertilization, or at implantation, or when the cerebral cortex is formed (at day 1 or day 120 after conception, or at birth?).[85]

In most developing countries, many of which have predominantly religious (Roman Catholic, Protestant, Islam, Hindu, Buddhist, etc.) communities, the trend is that abortion should not be a primary means of birth control; unwanted pregnancies are bound to occur, however, and it would be in the interest of women if facilities for obtaining abortions from qualified physicians were available. Abortion is accepted in China as a means of birth control and selective abortion is done after prenatal diagnosis of hemoglobin H disease, a mild to moderate thalassemic disease. Selective abortion following prenatal diagnosis of thalassemia is also an official policy in Cyprus, Greece, and Sardinia, but not in Thailand.[129]

It is not a policy in any part of black Africa to abort for the very common sickle-cell disease. Selective abortion on the basis of the sex of the fetus would be considered palpably wrong and unethical in most communities. Resorting to illegal abortion, a common practice when health care facilities are not available, carries enormous and significant risk to the life and health of women in developing countries. Most physicians in these countries would support the principle contained in the US Supreme Court decisions, *Webster v. Reproductive Health Services*, and *Roe v. Wade*, that it is a woman's right to decide whether to continue a pregnancy and that physicians and their patients have the freedom to make decisions about personal medical care.[7]

3. Contraceptive Devices
Family planning and population control are essential in developing countries, many of which have an annual growth rate of 3 percent or more (3.5 percent in Nigeria and 4 percent in Kenya). Opposition to the use of contraceptive devices is mainly religious, although some politicians in some developing countries naively believe that population control is not a priority. Physicians and health professionals who deliver family planning services have an obligation and duty to provide comprehensible information on the options available to couples. In many developing countries, it is inconceivable and unacceptable that a wife would resort to use of a contraceptive device without the knowledge (not necessarily the approval) of the husband.

Information should be given on the effectiveness and risks of the methods, although it has been argued[79] that in family planning, ethical conduct cannot always be equated with effective action. The use of contraceptive devices should be carefully monitored to detect and treat side-effects such as unusually heavy menstrual bleeding, amenorrhea, delayed return of menstruation and fertility after discontinuing use, significant weight gain, loss of libido, and depression and nervousness associated with the three monthly injections of Depo-provera. Incidentally, in spite of its world-wide use in over 90 countries, Depo-provera, manufactured and marketed by an American pharmaceutical organization, is not approved for use in the United States by the US Food and Drug Administration, and an accusation of "ethical double standards" has been made.[120] The French abortion pill RU 486, currently available only in France and China, has made it very easy for women to end pregnancies. Some regard the pill as a most welcome extension of women's reproductive choices. Others feel horrified at the ease with which women are allowed to end pregnancies.

It is ethical that population control be emphasized in developing countries as a requirement for progress in economic development and improved health conditions. Effective family planning and use of contraceptive devices are essential for population control. It is, in fact, an ethical imperative for the survival of the world.

Access of unmarried minors to family planning services and contraceptives without parental knowledge or consent is an ethical issue. In the context of most developing countries, sexual relationships outside marriage are frowned upon. Most parents would not consider it pious or proper to give consent to the use of contraceptives by children who are minors, and most parents would not, if pressed to make a decision, give such permission. It is worthy of note that as late as 1965, the state of Connecticut in the United States even prohibited married couples from using contraceptives.[7,43] In both developed and developing countries, there is a diversity of views about the permissibility of sexual relations between minors outside marriage. There is also uncertainty about when a minor should be granted the rights of an adult and what the extent of parental control of adolescent children might be. These issues are affected by myths about the consequences of parental notification. The status of minors and their rights, independent of parental control, remains unsettled in many societies.[79]

4. Fetal Tissue and Embryo Research

On ethical and religious grounds, many people oppose research using fetal tissue and human embryos, usually fertilized in vitro as part of an IVF/ET procedure or donated expressly for research by women undergoing sterilization. Fetal tissue for research is obtained as a result of elective abortion. Apart from the use of fetal tissue in transplantation (e.g. for treatment of Parkinson's disease or juvenile diabetes mellitus) the potential benefits of embryo research include: further development of infertility therapies; early prenatal diagnosis of genetic disorders; an increased understanding of reasons for miscarriages and the nature of chromosomal abnormalities.[46]

The most common objections to fetal tissue and embryo research include the following arguments:

1. The life of a human individual begins at conception with the fertilization of an ovum; it is wrong to kill human beings in order to carry out useful medical research.
2. Research with fetuses aborted electively is "ethically compromised" by the lack of authentic informed consent; it thereby offers the incentives for more abortions and increased complicity with abortion.
3. The aborting woman should not behave like a "devouring mother" but should fend off scavengers (the researchers) from the dead fetus.[6,89]

On the other hand, many others will not grant any embryo the moral recognition of a developing human life until after implantation. Hence in the United Kingdom, a fourteen-day limit on embryo research has been proposed, although a recent White paper, if accepted by Parliament, would outlaw embryo research altogether.[63] Sweden and the United States have also limited the period of research to fourteen days after fertilization. Intrauterine devices and progesterone-only contraceptive pills deprive embryos of a future just as much as research does. Therapeutic abortion destroys a fetus at a much more advanced stage of development than that of a pre-implantation embryo. It is difficult to justify the use of organs and tissues from dead children in transplantation without permitting the transplantation of tissues from dead fetuses.

With regard to the use of fetal tissue for transplantation, a U.S. Human Tissue Fetal Transplant Research Panel, created by the National Institutes of Health, made the following recommendation: "The decision to abort must be made before the tissue is discussed; anonymity should be maintained between donor and recipient, the timing and method of abortion should not be influenced by the potential use of the fetal tissues, and the consent of the pregnant woman is necessary and sufficient for use of tissue unless the father objects."[31] Some developing countries are capable of taking part in embryo and fetal tissue research, and a few have, in fact, done so. Neurosurgeons and researchers in Mexico, for instance, have used fetal transplants in the treatment of Parkinson's disease.[80] The ethical issues faced in developing countries and the attempts to solve them are similar.

ORGAN TRANSPLANTATION

Organ transplants in developing countries are relatively limited compared to the number which are done in developed countries.[1,92] For example, by 1984 less than 2 percent of the more than 100,000 kidney transplants carried out in the world had been done in developing countries.[1] The reason for this was mainly lack of resources, not reduced need. A kidney transplant costs more than US $30,000, and heart, liver, and lung transplants range between US $80,000 and US $100,000.[123] Principles of social justice and a utilitarian calculus would make it unlikely that the number of organ transplants would be increased in the near future in developing countries. From these perspectives, it would be unethical to allocate scarce resources for very expensive tertiary level intervention technology to benefit a relatively small group when primary health care for the vast majority could not be adequately funded and sustained.[1] In addition, cultural and religious beliefs, especially in the bodily existence of life after death, would prevent many people in certain parts of the developing world from agreeing to donate organs for transplantation. Islam does not prohibit organ donation or find it repugnant: in fact it supports it.[1]

In Ibadan, Nigeria, however, a corneal transplant program had to be abandoned because of lack of donors.[92] On the other hand, a number of Nigerians (especially mothers) have travelled abroad to serve as living donors for their children. For cadaver transplants, as in developed countries, the consent of relatives or of the deceased before death is required. In a number of developed countries, the sale of organs for transplantation by living donors is specified to be illegal. However, donation by competent adults of one of two paired organs (such as the kidney) whose removal does not significantly endanger the life of the donor is allowed, usually to a genetically or closely related recipient. Normally there are provisions to ensure that the donor has not been under any pressure of any kind.

The likelihood of living donors succumbing to the pressure of monetary inducement is great in developing countries. Recently, there have been increasing reports of instances in which residents of developing countries have been brought to developed countries in order to donate kidneys.[76] It has been argued that such donors are thereby able to raise money to do things for themselves or their families, a vital consideration. Such a consideration, they claim, would be an acceptable justification as it would mean that, ". . . a peasant could sell his kidney to stop his family from starving, a businessman to stop his factory closing, and even a student to pay for his education. . . . Ultimately the concept of motive would be abandoned and self-mutilation would become a commonplace last resort, but mutilation for profit would be unacceptable unlike mutilation for charity."[47]

The international trade in human organs, particularly live kidneys which usually pass from underdeveloped to developed countries, as well as the alleged practice of kidnapping and killing children for their organs, has been condemned in international fora.[32,39,40,132] Currently, a little over twenty countries--Canada, the United States, and most Western European countries--have legal provisions or policies which prohibit the sale of live organs. In July 1989, the United Kingdom enacted the Human Organ Transplant Act in response to sordid but true reports that many persons in Turkey and India were induced to sell their kidneys to wealthy recipients in London: the doctors involved were appropriately censored by the statutory professional body.[47]

The issue of when to declare a person dead so that life support systems may be switched off and organs may be removed for transplantation has aroused considerable debate over the past decade.[38,54,72,96,105] It would be useful to have an international consensus on the definition of brain death, as criteria vary internationally and even regionally (as within the United States).[38] Many countries such as the United Kingdom rely almost entirely on clinical criteria. Others such as Czechoslovakia and Sweden, for instance, require additional instrumental data (isoelectric EEG and arterial nonfilling of cerebral vasculature). Some countries including Denmark and the Islamic states do not accept brain death as synonymous with death. When a television program in one developed country (European) suggested erroneously in October 1980 that organs might be removed from donors who were not really dead (based on the opinion that brain death is not death), several potential donors withdrew their consent.

There is also the lesser, but important issue of definition of death in anencephalics: some have described the anencephalic state as "brain-absence" to enable the organs of these infants to be removed for transplantation while they are still technically alive.[122] Most developing countries (especially in sub-Saharan Africa, where organ transplantation is rarely performed) have not yet addressed the issue of definition of brain death.

SCREENING AND COUNSELING

The main thrust and objectives of screening are the achievement of early detection, the prevention and treatment of disease, and the promotion of health. In most developing countries where resources for health care are severely limited, cost-effectiveness and cost-benefit analysis are important to consider before the formulation of policies on screening. For instance, it could be relevant to know the number of quality-adjusted life years per unit of money spent in screening for cancer of the breast in a community as compared with the same assessment in a community with no screening at all. Information may not be available for such a community, and so extrapolation from other studies would have to be done. Research to answer such questions on cost-effectiveness should be started as soon as possible. In the United Kingdom it was estimated that screening for cervical and breast cancer cost £300,000 and £80,000 respectively per life saved and that screening was not affordable without incurring an inequitable and unethical distribution of the resources allocated to the national health services.[104,106] In the United States, a calculation was done in 1982 to determine whether yearly or tri-annual cervical smears should be done. The result obtained was that one would need to invest US $50,000 in additional cervical smears to prevent one more death from cancer.[74]

Screening tests, ideally, should be cheap, acceptable, valid, reliable, repeatable, sensitive, specific, and risk- free.[83] In British Columbia and in the United Kingdom, a common screening test such as a cervical smear to detect cervical carcinoma is thought to be unsatisfactory in most aspects and to have had little or no effect in reducing mortality and morbidity from cervical carcinoma.[87,124] In the United Kingdom, 40 million smears have been done. The pattern of falling mortality from cervical carcinoma observed in some developed countries appears to be independent of screening.[83] In addition, the screening test for cervical carcinoma is known to have harmful effects which include distress and anxiety created by false positive tests and cross infection. Yet in developing countries, this is one of the screening tests often recommended at least once every ten years for adult women aged 35-55.[118] It is ethically important to undertake more studies of the cost-effectiveness of screening for cervical carcinoma in developing countries.

In determining health policy on screening, an important consideration is the feasibility of treatment and prevention of the condition for which screening is being done. It would be unethical to screen for hypertension in a population in which the frequency of hypertension is 10 percent or more (as obtains in most developing countries in Africa) when all who are hypertensive and require treatment cannot be offered adequate health care. From a study at Ibadan, Nigeria, the compliance for treatment is very poor in those who are asymptomatic hypertensive. Screening for sickle cell trait, present in 25 percent of black populations in Africa, would also be unrewarding in term of cost-effectiveness.

In the last decade, with the rapid advances in molecular biology and genetics, screening for prenatal diagnosis of some genetic diseases has become an important part of established good medical practice. In some circumstances, if the facilities are available, it would be unethical not to screen, especially those known to be carriers or to have a positive family history or some well-known risk factors such as advanced maternal age. In developed countries there already have been instances of those born with a disability who have sued their parents for negligence in allowing them to have been born, as well as parents who have prosecuted physicians for failure to advise on the possibility of prenatal testing or for negligence in performing it.[60] The objective of prenatal diagnosis is threefold: .

1. To detect abnormalities in utero with the aim of correcting them where possible;
2. To carry out selective abortion for untreatable conditions; and
3. To provide information to couples opposed to abortion so that the couple may plan for a child with a disability.

Prenatal diagnosis also offers an opportunity to reassure the mother if the fetus is normal and to obtain information that would be useful in the management of the pregnancy and birth. Ethical questions relate to:

1. Whether abortion should be done for all abnormalities or only the serious ones;
2. Whether abortion should be done for abnormalities detected after the fetus is viable; and
3. Whether prenatal diagnosis should be carried out in a woman who is opposed to abortion.

The important thing is that a complete discussion of these issues should be held with the woman or couple. The choices and options should be clearly agreed upon before the diagnostic procedure is begun, and full informed consent must be always obtained.

Selective abortion on the basis of the sex of a fetus would be unethical and unacceptable in most developing countries, even though males are often preferred. There is some evidence that in certain countries such as India and China[29] selective abortion on the basis of sex is practiced illegally and frequently, especially in families with a preponderance of female offspring (in India) or to ensure that the one child officially allowed by government policy is a male (China).

There is the problem of HIV infection and AIDS and the related ethical issue as to whether pregnant women should be routinely screened for HIV infection. I share the view that, on this issue, pregnant women should not be treated differently from other members of society. Unless screening for HIV infection is compulsory for all in a particular community, it should be carried out on pregnant women, if at all, only with their informed consent and under conditions of confidentiality.[12]

MAPPING AND SEQUENCING OF THE HUMAN GENOME: ETHICAL ISSUES ON USE AND MISUSE

The resources and organization of several institutions have been mobilized over the past three or four years with the aim of achieving within the next fifteen years what has been likened to a "moon-shot" in molecular biology.[101] Their aim is the sequencing of the 3.5 billion nucleotide base pairs in human 46 chromosomes and the mapping (location of genes on chromosomes) of the human genome. The institutions currently involved in this US $3 billion project are all in the developed countries (United States, Europe, and Japan). Of the estimated 50,000 to 100,000 genes in the human genome, some 4,600 are already known. Of those known, 1,500 have been mapped to specific chromosomes and 600 or more have been cloned.[84] Although there is still a long way to go, it seems likely that the task will be achieved once the required technological tools are fully developed. Everyone is agreed that mapping and sequencing of the human genome will not "unlock the secrets of life."[101]

The payoff from gene mapping and sequencing has already begun, as shown by valuable contributions to clinical medicine. In the past decade several important Mendelian disorders have been mapped. These include hereditary sensory motor neuropathy on chromosome 1, Huntington's disease on chromosome 4, adenomatous polyposis of colon on chromosome 5, cystic fibrosis on chromosome 7, tuberous sclerosis and idiopathic torsion dystonia in Ashkenazi Jews on chromosome 9, retinoblastoma on chromosome 16, peripheral type of neurofibromatosis on chromosome 17 and central type on chromosome 22, dystrophia myotonica on chromosome 19, one form of familial Alzheimer's disease on chromosome 21, Duchenne's muscular dystrophy (DMD) and its Becker variant on the short arm of X chromosome. Prenatal diagnosis of some of these diseases such as DMD, neurofibromatosis, and cystic fibrosis is now possible. Premorbid diagnosis and carrier detection of diseases such as Huntington's disease is now well established. It is possible now in some diseases such as DMD to identify the nature of the lesion of the gene and to describe the effects which produce the disease: this could guide the development of forms of therapy including gene therapy or gene modification (i.e. somatic gene therapy which is not fundamentally different from organ transplantation or blood transfusion).[51]

Diseases which might be treated with gene therapy will be exclusively single-gene disorders in which the expression of the normal gene is not very complex. Preferred candidates for gene therapy would be patients with diseases which are invariably fatal or severely incapacitating and for whom there are no safe, effective current therapies.[51] Gene mapping and sequencing presents enormous potentiality in improved understanding of carcinogenesis, identification of the specific genomic changes as the fundamental cause or mechanism of abnormal growth, and in control of diseases including cancer and even mental illness. The mapping and sequencing of the human genome has been described as a "new anatomy . . . neo-Vesalian basis for medicine of decades to come."[84]

Abuse of the mapping and sequencing of the human genome might include misuse of information about an individual's genetic abnormality to deny employment or insurance[51,94] and misuse in eugenics, i.e., as the basis for genetic selection through modification or insertion of genes into germ cells (germline cell therapy) in order to create "special" humans through enhancement of general characteristics such as physical appearance or intelligence.[50,51] As a method of treatment, attention has been focused on the use of retroviruses as vectors for the introduction of genes into cells.[51,115] There is always the risk that the vector virus may not be sufficiently disabled and so may subsequently replicate, hence posing a finite risk of viral escape.[127] The retrovirus is usually packaged with the aid of a "helper" virus and this must be totally removed from the vector preparations. The inserted gene, the helper, and the vector viruses might activate the expression of genes involved in the induction of cancer or induce oncogenes, or it might cause other harmful disturbances of cell regulation or function.[51] The inserted gene might also spread into other cells, including germ cells.

It is obvious that gene therapy will be experimental for a number of years and the usual guidelines on research involving human subjects must apply. Being new, gene therapy would only be justifiable in invariably fatal or life-threatening diseases where no alternative therapy is available. It would also be essential to ensure that both the safety and efficacy of such a novel therapy are clearly determined and defined.

I subscribe to the view of the European Medical Research Council that germ-line therapy should not be contemplated or embarked upon.[51] It is disturbing that a reputable scientific medical journal reacted to this viewpoint as follows: "Why not? How different are the decisions that parents now take that affect their offspring to those that involve inserting genes into the germline. Women choose the fathers of their children. They may choose to have children knowing that they have a high chance of having a genetic defect: they usually do so knowingly. If mothers have the right to bear children with AIDS why can they not choose to have a genetic defect corrected and so not pass it on to their children."[50] No one will challenge the right of women to have a genetic defect corrected, but this may develop into a slippery slope on which germ-line therapy, once begun as a practice, opens the way to many types of abuse. Monsters and super-race humans could be produced. The myths created by Mary Shelley's Dr. Frankenstein, H.G. Wells' Dr. Moreau, and the minotaur (the hybrid creation of King Minos' wife and a bull)[50] could become real.

Some people wonder how it is possible that people are frightened of genetic engineering.[50] However, to many the fear is genuine. So it is necessary to provide education and information about procedures and possibilities and to set up national regulatory bodies as advised by the European Medical Research Councils. It is true "that the technical aspects of gene therapy are complex, the issues moderately simple and that there are no grand new ethical considerations,"[50] but the norms of existing ethical guidelines must be kept. If there were to be any biological disaster resulting from gene experimentation, the whole world could be involved.

LIVING AND DYING:
EUTHANASIA AND CRITICAL CARE MEDICINE

In most extant cultures in the developing countries (whether or not influenced by imported religion--Judeo-Christianity and Islam, mainly), life is regarded as sacred, of supreme value and inestimable worth. Both Islam and

Judeo-Christianity enjoin that preservation of life is a divine order: Judeo-Christianity urges "thou shalt not kill" and Islam prescribes that the unlawful slaying of a single soul will be equivalent to the killing of all mankind. No one is entitled to commit any direct or indirect action that would destroy his or her own or anyone else's life--an injunction common to all the great religions.[2,98,102,117] In Buddhism, the religion of millions in Southeast Asia, death is an integral part of existence and is one phase of an endless cycle. Buddhism prohibits suicide and the taking of life for any reason including painful and incurable disease because such an action is an obstacle to the attainment of nirvana, the highest Buddhist ideal.[102] On the other hand, there is what has been described as secular humanism (which specifies that mankind is not subject to moral rules or principles that have a supernatural origin), a movement of ancient origin not related to atheism or to existentialism. Secular humanism is, in part, based on the teaching of the pre-Socratic philosopher Protagoras that "man is the measure of all things." This implies that decisions and conclusions are made on the basis of human judgment and not on a theology or religion-based morality.[56] The attitude of the secular humanist regarding the end of life is therefore different from that of those who believe in theology and religion. Secular humanism, of course, is not prevalent in developing countries.

In Jewish philosophy, death is inevitable and makes way for new life and continued creation.[117] The Christian view is not dissimilar in that it sees death as necessarily prior to redemption by the living God. It allows for victory over sin and an entry into the world beyond which will be, for the just, a sharing in the life of Christ.[98] Both Judeo-Christianity and Islam prohibit euthanasia, although in Christianity, as called for by Job and Christ, divine help may be sought to relieve or to end the agony of dying or suffering. Buddhism teaches that quality of life is more important than its duration.[102]

Many Africans are very stoical in their traditional beliefs about suffering, due to the belief that it comes from the Almighty or some of the Almighty's servants, or from an offended ancestral spirit, a wicked sorcerer, or witch. Attempts are made to placate the causal agent by offering a sacrifice after consulting the diviner or taking appropriate measures to counteract the effects of sorcery or witchcraft. The death of an elderly person, especially if survived by children, is celebrated with pomp, as are births and marriages. Suicide is relatively rare, although death is preferred to dishonor, especially in order to preserve a family's good name. Most Africans believe there is a clear-cut difference between living and existing. Euthanasia (not by health personnel but by relations) was and is probably widely practiced unofficially in the African culture for incurable and distressful mental illness and severe congenital malformations.[91]

In most developing countries, euthanasia is hardly ever discussed because its concept is more or less repugnant and the implementation of it unthinkable. Active euthanasia by doctors is contrary to the basic principles of the medical profession. Doctors serve their patients best by accurate prognosis and skillful management of pain and complications.[62] In addition, the practices of active euthanasia, if encouraged, might be abused. An eminent contemporary philosopher, R.M. Hare writes: "Doctors would do well, having adopted some fairly simple set of principles which copes adequately with the cases they are likely to meet, to dismiss from their minds (at least when they are doctoring) the possibility of there being further exceptions to their principles. For doctors, like all of us, are human. If once they start thinking when engaged on a case, that this case might be one of the limitless and indeterminate set of exceptions to their principles, they will find such exceptions everywhere."[20]

In developing countries, aimless and endless prolongation of life by technological means does not usually happen. This is compatible with the culture of the peoples and the teachings of the great religions--Judeo-Christianity, Islam, and Buddhism.[2,61,98,102] The British Medical Association, after full consideration of the report of a working committee, rejected euthanasia.[20,90] Of course, the developing countries must keep *au fait* with current thinking on euthanasia and related issues. It is important to be aware of the dialogues and developing codes concerning living wills, do-not-resuscitate (DNR) orders, durable power of attorney for health care, ethical principles in critical care medicine, and the pro-euthanasia movement, especially in Europe and particularly in the Netherlands.[37,90] It should be pointed out that in a country such as the United States, some of the practices that were controversial five years ago in the care of the dying patient have now become accepted routine.[71,128]

Living wills are now respected, and DNR orders are acceptable if made by competent patients (with unimpaired decisionmaking capacity) or surrogates. Both the common law right to autonomy (to be left alone to make one's choice) and the right to privacy (to be protected from unwanted invasive medical treatment) are now recognized. Near total relief of pain and discomfort is justifiable even if it accelerates the demise of the patient.[128] It is now accepted that there is little or no difference between nasogastric or intravenous hydration and other life-sustaining measures which could be withdrawn in hopelessly ill patients on demand, by competent patients, family, or surrogates.[77,88] A doctor must not substitute his or her decision for that of the patient's validly made choice.[18] The basic principles of medical ethics, particularly that of respect for persons through informed consent, must be honored. It must be realized that human life is more than a biological process which must be supported in all situations. As noted by the poet Clough, "Thou shall not kill, but do not officiously strive to keep alive." The principle of fairness or social justice obligates physicians to avoid the waste of limited resources on patients who cannot be helped.[77] It would be ideal if, in the near future, international guidelines could be formulated regarding when to forego or withdraw medical treatment. A good beginning has been made by a group of thirty-three physicians, bioethicists, and medical economists from ten different sets of cultural conditions who met at the University of Appleton in Lawrence, Wisconsin (USA), to develop the Appleton consensus.[116]

CARE OF THE ELDERLY

Health care for the elderly is going to assume an increasing importance in the near future, both in developed countries where the proportion of the population over the age of sixty-five (the elderly) is of the order of 10 to 15 percent or more, and in the developing countries where, because of large populations, the actual numbers of elderly are extremely high. Of course, the increase in the number of people reaching old age is a success story due to improvement in nutrition; to environmental, food, and water sanitation; to reduction in childhood mortality; and to improved means of prevention and treatment of diseases. Currently, of the 370 million elderly people in the world, 52 percent live in the developing countries. Worldwide, there is a monthly increase of 1.2 million elderly. Of these elderly, 80 percent live in the developing countries. By 2025 AD the numbers of elderly will have increased to 1 billion, and 75 percent of them will live in developing countries. It is obvious that very soon the problems of the elderly, and of the longevity revolution, will be taxing the resources of the developing countries. Most of these countries are undergoing epidemiological transition and the organization of social services is either very rudimentary or non-existent. In developing countries the extended family system, which has traditionally provided a buffer in the care of the elderly, is being remorselessly dismantled.[92]

In most developing countries, the elderly are normally much loved, respected, and valued, and they are cared for by the entire family. They are not looked upon as being non-productive and hence not worthy of care. However, social and health care infrastructure in most parts of the developing world does not adequately provide for support of the elderly or for solving their medical, mental, and socioeconomic problems. The elderly often have to depend on their children and other members of the family. Currently, in most developing countries, prevalence of dementias of the elderly, and particularly of primary dementias of Alzheimer's type (which accounts for 50 to 60 percent of the dementias of the elderly in developed countries, apart from Japan) is low compared with the situation in the developed countries.[93] The cost of care for the elderly who are demented is very high, especially in societies where institutional care is the rule rather than the exception. For example, in the United States the cost of institutional care for patients with dementia was estimated in 1985 to exceed US $25 billion, or more than 5 percent of the total cost of national care.[68] Osteoporosis with hip fractures and ischemic heart disease are also less common in the elderly in developing countries than in developed countries.

As a social justice and equality concern, health policy in the developing world ought to take into account the burgeoning health care needs of the elderly, both with and without the support of the family. There is no such policy in most developing countries. It is disturbing to know that an age-based limitation on medical care is being considered in some countries in the developed world.[20] With this criterion, for instance, anyone could propose denial of certain health care facilities to those over the age of sixty-five.[73] Of course, one can justify ethically the concept of health care rationing in the face of limited resources. This implies certain deliberate choices about the sharing of health care resources among persons, such as who gets what care and in what order of priority and on what grounds. The grounds, when social justice is being considered, go beyond an individual patient's clinically defined needs and include consideration of comparative medical need and social equity.[103] It would appear, however, that the main rationale for jettisoning anyone off the "lifeboat" must not be age, for that would be unethical: rights of people are not dependent on age.[123] The elderly belong to a group that deserves gratitude for its past contributions, since they are largely responsible for any country's prosperity and survival. Of course, appropriate balancing must be done in allocating and rationing resources. If most elderly people in developing countries were asked today whether they would favor their children and grandchildren or themselves in the allocation of resources for health care, the answer would undoubtedly be that they prefer that more resources go to the children and their mothers. This is a choice also favored by some in the United Kingdom.[16]

In developing countries, the quality of life of the elderly is considered very important. They are well cared for according to the ability of the family and with the best affordable facilities, but unnecessarily heroic measures which painfully prolong dying are avoided.

In developed countries, some of the expenditure on health care for the elderly is six times that spent on the health of those under the age of eighteen,[21] it has been necessary to attempt to define health care policy for the elderly. The same is needed in developing countries. This would spell out what could be done to ensure that "old age, as the beginning of a new life," is lived happily and productively without suffering and pain, and within the limits of available resources. As much as possible every encouragement should be given to the extended family system so that it is preserved for as long as possible. Families who look after their elderly could, for example, be adequately compensated from public funds. There would be a need to establish facilities to provide institutional and community care for the elderly in the developing countries.

Work is one of the greatest promoters of health. The practice of compulsory retirement of "elderly" people in the developed countries could be reviewed where it would not accentuate unemployment. In many developing countries, people retire between fifty-five years and sixty-five years. Age alone should not be a criterion for retirement, at least before seventy years as now occurs in some developed countries: the important criterion should be functional capacity to perform the appropriate tasks and duties.

Developing countries could also borrow from the experience of some developed countries where the elderly, as senior citizens, are given special rights such as reduced transport fares and exemption from payment of certain fees.

So far, public health policies in most developing countries have relatively neglected the health care of the elderly. This is certainly unethical, and it is time that this oversight is corrected.

USE AND MISUSE OF TECHNOLOGY

Currently the most widely blamed culprit for the upward spiralling cost of health care in a number of developed countries is the excessive, unnecessary, and irrelevant use of technology, that is, the apparatus and procedures that are based on modern science. There are also other causes such as waste, inefficiency, clumsy and expensive bureaucratic systems, over-consumption by the public of care that is virtually free because of prepayment or previous taxation, and overuse by health personnel (especially doctors) for personal gain.[82] It is said that in developed countries, technology has seduced the medical profession.[82] Most members of the medical profession are driven by a stubborn desire for diagnostic certainty through excessive use of diagnostic tests[82] which, in turn, are often based on sophisticated technology. Causes of excessive testing include inordinate zeal for complete diagnostic certainty, pressure from peers and supervisors, the convenience with which tests are ordered, the demands of the patient or family, and the desire to avoid malpractice claims.[67] One estimate suggests that in a developed country such as the United States, diagnostic tests involving the use of expensive machines, radioisotopes, electronics, and imaging techniques, consumed 50 percent of the current annual health care bill of over US $500 billion. There is also the use and misuse of what has been called therapeutic technology, i.e. complex surgical and intervention procedures such as organ transplants; installation of expensive devices such as pacemakers; procedures requiring expensive equipment such as radiotherapy, lithotripsy, or dialysis; use of expensive drugs, such as recombinant produced erythropoietin, or tissue plasminogen activator (TPA, which currently costs US $1,200 per treatment).

The benefit to patients of these new technologies is clear in many cases. Conservative management of acute myocardial infarction with intravenous recombinant TPA, heparin, and aspirin without coronary arteriography and angioplasty has saved US $200 million annually.[118] In some instances, however, the treatments are of dubious value, fully untried or untested, or less cost-effective compared with not-so-new or with older technologies. The interest of developing countries in these technologies rises, quite often, before they have been adequately tried and tested for cost-effectiveness.

Technological "advances" are "transferred" to the developing countries, whose physicians are "encouraged" by sales forces to recommend their acquisition to decisionmakers. One is reminded of the early days of coronary bypass surgery, in which it took nearly ten years and more than 400,000 operations at a cost of US $50 billion before it was realized that only a subset of patients--those with left main coronary or three vessel disease--significantly benefitted from the operation in terms of quality of life and survival. Developing countries have severely limited resources for health care compared with developed countries, and they should spend these resources in a fair manner, from a social justice perspective based on sound principles of health economics.

Ideally, the developing countries should set up national review committees for evaluating technologies before purchase. However, this is not always possible. Before acquisition, new technologies for health care systems should be carefully evaluated for their potential benefits and costs. Such a cost-benefit analysis for these technologies could then be compared with a cost-effectiveness analysis for available existing technologies. The United States Health Care Financing Administration, which manages the Medicare program, has suggested the following cost-effectiveness criteria:

● The new technology must be less expensive and at least as effective as any extant alternative technology.
● If it is more expensive than an alternative, it must also be more effective and bring about improved outcomes to justify the additional expense.
● If it is less effective and less expensive than an alternative, it should be used if it is viable for some patients.

HIV INFECTION AND THE AIDS PANDEMIC

The epidemic of human immunodeficiency virus (HIV) infection causing acquired immune deficiency syndrome (AIDS) is a transnational disease from which no society will be completely protected without global control. The ethical issues are myriad. I wish only to refer to a few aspects.

AIDS was first described in the United States in 1981, and the HIV virus was identified in 1983. AIDS was not described in black Africa until 1983. By December 31, 1989, some 5 to 10 million people were believed to be infected and 203,599 cases including 38,248 cases from Africa had been reported to the WHO. Most of the African cases were from Central and East African countries. By far the majority of the total cases reported have come from the United States: in only two years, 1988 and 1989, there were reported 32,196 and 35,238 cases, respectively.[24] In spite of a lack of hard scientific evidence, Western scientists speculated that HIV might have originated in Africa, and the distribution of Kaposi's sarcoma, a malignancy frequently associated with AIDS, was held to be strong evidence for this hypothesis.[112] It is now believed that Kaposi's sarcoma is caused by a transmissible agent other than HIV.[15,41] Although the misinformation about the African origin has been shown to be unlikely to be true,[70,108] the inaccuracies persist: Africans continue to be stigmatized as carriers of HIV. This, to me, appears to be unethical and totally unjust. Couldn't the medical profession make a special appeal to the Western press to be more responsible, so as not to create a negative, anti-research, AIDS-does-not-occur-in-our-country attitude among African countries?

Surely quarantine is not the solution to the HIV pandemic, as the median incubation period between infection and AIDS could be as long as ten years. Where would you quarantine the approximately 5 million people who are already infected? The medical profession should speak out more convincingly against countries who have embarked on a quarantine of seropositive individuals. Other forms of discrimination (such as restriction on travel and refusal of entry in certain countries and denial of access to schools) have been suffered by HIV seropositive individuals and AIDS patients. Unlinked anonymous screening for public health surveillance is ethically just.[8] Compulsory testing is discriminatory and assaults privacy. Some have argued that this is necessary for people such as airline pilots who hold sensitive public safety positions.

Two meetings, one in 1988 and the second in 1990, sponsored by the World Health Organization reviewed the results of some eleven investigations on the functional status of asymptomatic seropositives and found disagreement as to whether abnormalities as measured by neuropsychological testing occurred with increased frequency in otherwise healthy HIV-1 infected persons.[133,134] The 1990 meeting concluded that the frequency of functional impairment is not significantly increased (over the levels found in HIV-1 uninfected people) until or unless patients became ill with AIDS related complex or AIDS. The earlier meeting in 1988 had pointed out that the critical issue was not the cause of impaired job performance. It was, instead, the ability to detect impairment, whatever the cause, for a vast number of conditions that may prevent adequate performance. These limiting conditions include stress, fatigue, disruption of circadian rhythms, aging, substance abuse, and psychiatric disorders. A recent paper published after the 1990 WHO meeting reported results which suggest that cognitive inefficiency occurred in a sub-sample of individuals during early HIV infection.[126] So far, the studies of asymptomatic HIV-1 seropositive individuals in which no increase of the frequency of abnormal neuropsychological findings have been demonstrated included a total of more than 1,100 subjects, while the studies showing such an increase included a total of 309 subjects. The weight of currently available evidence suggests that otherwise healthy HIV infected individuals are not more likely to be functionally impaired than persons uninfected with HIV-1. Hence there is at the present time no justification for HIV-1 serological screening of asymptomatic persons as a strategy for detecting such functional impairment in the interest of public safety. There is a need to review this conclusion in the light of studies currently in progress or planned. So far, homosexual or bisexual men in industrialized countries have been the only subjects for these. The conclusion may also not apply to other risk groups with different levels of education or with different frequencies of confounding factors such as the use of alcohol and other drugs.[133,134]

AIDS and HIV infection have raised issues concerning conflicts between the civil rights of individuals and the needs of communities and societies, and they have brought to awareness the question of how to protect lives without violating and nullifying basic civil rights and freedoms.[75,99] Unless individuals respond adequately to health education by responsible behavior modification to help control spread of the epidemic, the welfare of the community or society will take precedence over the rights of individuals. This ethical consideration may relate to an infected individual who will not use a condom, to infected prostitutes, to an infected individual who has a spouse, and to infected intravenous drug users who insist on sharing needles. The government may need to play a greater role than normally would be the case, since the needs of the community must be given a certain priority when it is a matter of life and death and the spread of a fatal disease. Nevertheless, great caution and vigilance are needed to protect individual freedoms as much as possible.

Many developing countries, because of lack of resources are unable to screen all blood units for transfusion. Is it ethical in these circumstances to transfuse unscreened blood? Who pays compensation to those who receive infected blood? Some developed countries pay compensation to hemophiliacs who were infected before HIV was detected; others do not pay. Most developing countries cannot afford to pay. What about the infected health professional? Does he go on practicing? What about the health professional who will not treat an AIDS or HIV seropositive individual? That would be unethical: the practices of medicine and nursing have always carried their own risks and hazards.[94]

AIDS challenges many aspects of conventional medical practice, societal ethics, and control and disposition of resources[3] for a disease which currently has no cure. Should developing countries, where the annual per capita expenditure on health is US $1.00 to US $5.00, invest in treatment of AIDS or HIV carriers with zidovudine, when the annual cost of treatment is currently over US $6,000? To most developing countries in Africa, purchase of zidovudine from public funds for treatment of AIDS or asymptomatic HIV subjects is out of the question. AIDS challenges the basic concepts of intimate relationship and makes the citizenship vulnerable: the disease might alter the value placed on individual freedom and change the normal or accepted views of fairness, and equality.[99] Certainly AIDS has modified views about autonomy, consent, and confidentiality in all countries, both developed and developing.[34] An impressive bibliography on ethical issues in AIDS has been compiled[81] referencing documents related to:

- Measures taken by governments to protect society. These include quarantine and isolation, discriminatory measures directed at specific groups, lack of respect for the confidential nature of medical information, application of the penal code, screening, obligatory declaration and registration, testing of blood given by donors, vaccination and medical innovations, therapeutic assays, and information and education.
- Measures intended to protect the individual. These include protection of the fundamental rights of patients as follows:
  - Rights to confidentiality, to information, and to treatment;
  - Civil rights, including rights to civil liberty, education, and work;
  - Rights of the healthy individual, including those in contact with the patients including safety of hospital staff and recipients of blood transfusions.

Protective measures may also include certain types of legislation adopted in various countries. It is worthy of note that no country in sub-Saharan Africa has legislated on any issue related to AIDS and HIV infection.

There are also ethical issues related to the testing of HIV vaccines. Such testing must conform to the accepted guidelines on biomedical ethics in research involving human subjects. These have been referenced previously.

ALTERNATIVE MEDICINE OR HEALTH CARE SYSTEMS IN DEVELOPING COUNTRIES

In many developing countries, a high proportion of the population use the procedures of alternative medicine. In sub-Saharan Africa, it is possible that as many as 80 percent of black Africans resort to traditional medicine, either as the only form of health care available (especially in the rural areas) or in combination with Western medicine. Ayurveda, which is literally translated as science of life, developed as a system of medicine in India more than 2,000 years ago, and is still widely used. Acupuncture has now spread beyond China, and some of its effectiveness, such as relief of pain through release of endogenous endorphins, has been found to have a scientific rationale. I believe, for ethical reasons, including the honoring of justice and equality, as well as utilitarian considerations, that alternative medicine systems should not be ignored. They should be thoroughly investigated so that their positive aspects can be assimilated into health care services and their harmful practices discarded. After all, the alternative health care systems in developing countries have provided modern Western medicine with effective drugs such as quinine, physostigmine, reserpine, rauwolfia alkaloids and reserpine, vincristine, quinghaosu (artemisia annua), and feverfew, to mention a few.

In many developing countries in Africa, in spite of the ubiquity of traditional native practitioners, no attempt is made to control and regulate their practice. I believe this is unethical, for some of them are charlatans and untrained and many frequently traduce one of the basic principles of medical ethics, nonmaleficience or *primum non nocere*. For example, in some parts of Nigeria, the hands and feet of a patient in post-epileptic unconsciousness are thrust into a fire and pepper is put into the conjunctival sac in a vain attempt to wake him. The result is severe burns and contractures and corneal injuries with blindness. In other cases, psychotic patients are shackled with iron chains which often inflict severe trauma.

In my view, it is also ethical to evaluate traditional medicine in various communities by means of the quantification and numerate methods of biostatistics and clinical epidemiology. If developing countries are to make serious efforts to integrate traditional medicine into the health care delivery system, then these ethical issues must be looked into. In many developing countries, traditional medicine cannot be replaced entirely by Western medicine. Unlike Western medicine, traditional medicine is a comprehensive aggregate of ideas, beliefs, and practices relating not only to medicine, but also to magic, religion, and a societal way of life.[91] It is relevant to mention that various forms of alternative medicine still coexist with traditional Western medicine in most developed countries. Even distinguished royalty has strongly favored the use of alternative medical systems.[46]

POLITICAL ABUSE OF MEDICINE

In a few countries, health policies have recently been applied to punish political opponents, as well as to reward political supporters. There have also been direct involvement of health personnel in political or punitive acts which contradicted accepted medical ethical practices.[86,136] Health care personnel have been tyrannized and threatened with punishment including execution, for no other reasons than that they spoke out or acted in favor of their clientele. Suppression of important health information, as has happened in countries which initially denied the existence of AIDS so as not to jeopardize international tourism,[55] also amounts to political abuse of medicine and is unethical. It is imperative that the health care professions in other countries should speak out when there has been political abuse of medicine in any country.

ADVERTISING

The cultural response of many communities in most developing countries to advertisement by health personnel, especially by physicians, will be amazement, surprise, disbelief, and disgust. Physicians are held in high respect, and are thought to be omniscient beings second only to the Almighty.[91] All professional medical regulatory bodies in developing countries prohibit advertisement by physicians. Advertisement by health personnel would damage the reputation of the health professions and could be abused. False claims giving false hopes could have disastrous and irrevocable consequences for patients.

It is noted that in some developed countries, especially the United Kingdom, it is being considered or proposed that certain categories of physicians, such as general practitioner, should be allowed to advertise subject to certain safeguards. The advertisement should not be of a character that could be regarded as likely to bring the profession into disrepute. It should not be such as to abuse the trust of patients or potential patients or exploit their lack of knowledge. The advertisement should be factual, legal, decent, honest, and truthful. It should not disparage other doctors or make claims of superiority. It should not explicitly or implicitly claim to cure particular illnesses.[28,53]

I believe the ethos of most health care personnel in the developing countries support the assertion that the motives of health care professionals are, by and large, altruistic ones and that such altruism is not to be marketed. The health professions, particularly the medical profession, should abide by the principles of learned professions and of the professional societies which ban advertising. It is said[78] that nine features distinguish a learned profession from others:

- Service to the poor without expectation of compensation
- Quality service
- Reasonable fees
- High level of education and training
- Autonomy of activity
- Altruism with certain threadbare nobility
- Self-sacrifice
- Heroism as needed
- Ethical practice with public accountability

Profitmaking is not central to medicine and the health care professions, at least in the developing countries. In these countries [unlike what has been proposed by one developed country],[45] health care should not be marketed as a commodity.

INDUSTRIAL/PHARMACEUTICAL MARKETING AND MEDICAL ETHICS

A recent trend in developed countries is the involvement of health care personnel in advertising or promotion of products from the industrial/pharmaceutical industry in return for a favor given in kind or cash or some other form of compensation. This practice is also creeping into the developing countries. Some of the industrial/pharmaceutical organizations involved also support health research. As has been pointed out, "The profession of medicine and the industries that provide the products needed for patient care and research are by nature interdependent. A large part of both clinical and basic research is funded by the companies that produce pharmaceuticals, supplies for patient care, complex diagnostic and therapeutic machinery, prosthetic devices and other indispensable materials."[19]

Both the industrial/pharmaceutical industry and the health care profession need to maintain a good ethical relationship for the benefit of health care recipients. Although physicians may wish to benefit from the relationship, the acceptance of significant favors and enticements is unethical and carries the risk of bias and loss of objectivity. In addition, the costs of these enticements to the industrial/pharmaceutical organizations are unfairly passed on to the consumers. I believe that personal remuneration to physicians from a pharmaceutical organization for bringing patients into a clinical trial is not ethically justifiable.[107]

CONCLUSION

Biomedical ethical issues, guidelines, principles, and regulations cut across national boundaries and often have universal implications. Peoples differ and so do cultures, but certain values are common to all. In this context, the most important value is respect for human dignity, and this should not be negotiable.

In many developing countries there is no mechanism for management of research. For example, only twenty-two out of forty-five countries in black Africa have medical research councils or equivalents. Only a few of those that have medical research councils also have national ethical committees or equivalents. Institutional ethical committees in medical schools and research institutes in developing countries are often ineffective. In many developing countries there are no equivalents of the U.S. Food and Drug Administration setup and the control it exercises. Most, however, have professional statutory regulatory bodies which also perform some functions such as being the ethical watchdog for professional ethical behavior.

It is important that every country have a dynamic mechanism for dealing with ethical problems as well as for regulating ethical norms in medical practice and research. Such a mechanism must be responsive to changes within and without the country and must take into consideration the views of the majority of the citizens.[35] It may involve the establishment of a national medical ethics commission and of regional, local, and institutional ethics committees. The national medical ethics commission would be responsible for formulating national policies on ethics in medical practice and research and would also evaluate for approval all externally funded or sponsored research projects: it should have access to lawmakers and the highest policymakers in the ministry of health.

For many developing countries that are frog-leaping centuries in development and undergoing epidemiological transition, conflicts in the constant flux of life do occur, frequently creating ethical problems, particularly against a background of rapid changes in Western medical and technological knowledge. Resolution is not impossible, once the necessary legal, administrative, political, and health care mechanisms are established. For example, traditional medicine does not need to be abolished, but it should be evaluated, and it would be highly unethical not to do so if the majority of a community continues to use the services.

Ethical guidelines should be dynamic, and they ought to be periodically reviewed. Ethical principles should be more like statutes, difficult to change. It should also be realized that in this jet age, communities do change, become deculturated, and acculturated. Obedience to tribal leaders[4] has disappeared in some communities within a generation. In many developing countries, political emancipation and periodic exposure to vote-seeking harangues have changed perception of collective leadership and of the role of the individual in the society and community. People are becoming increasingly better educated and more amenable to change, resulting in changing cultural habits. Human rights should be inviolable, but they are meant to be used to serve the society, and when they cease to do so or they are used to threaten the society, society has the right to protect itself. The duty of the health care professional is both to the society and to the patient, but he or she must first comply with the ethical principles that regulate the relationship between the health care giver and the consumer. The main thrust of biomedical ethics in health and research is to preserve human dignity and to implement social justice, thereby maintaining the good reputation of the health care professions.

NOTES

1   Abdussalam, M. "Organ Substitution Therapy in the Developing World: From Corneal Grafting to Renal Dialysis." In: Bankowski, Z., Bryant, J.H., eds. *Health Policy, Ethics and Human Values*. Geneva: CIOMS, 1985, p. 217-225.
2   Abul-Fadl, M.A.M. "Islam, History, Traditions, and Faith-Impacts on Health Policy Formulation." In: Bankowski, A., Bryant, J.H., eds. *Health Policy, Ethics, and Human Values*. Geneva: CIOMS, 1985, 87-95.
3   "AIDS: Prevention, Policies and Prostitutes." *Lancet* 1989, 1: 1111-1113.
4   Ajayi, O.O. "Taboos and Clinical Research in West Africa." *Journal of Medical Ethics* 1980, 6: 61-63.
5   Angell, M. "Ethical Imperialism? Ethics in International Collaborative Clinical Research." *New England Journal of Medicine* 1988, 319: 1081-1083.
6   Annas, G.J., Elias, S. "The Politics of Transplantation of Human Fetal Tissue." *New England Journal of Medicine* 1989, 320: 1079-1082.
7   Annas, G.J., Glantz, L.H., Wendy, K., Mariner, W.K. "The Right of Privacy Protects the Doctor-Patient Relationship." *Journal of the American Medical Association* 1990, 263: 858-861.
8   "Anonymous HIV Testing." *Lancet* 1990, 1: 575-576.
9   Ayitteh, G.B.N. "Helping Africans, Not By AID Alone." *International Herald Tribune* April 1990, 10.
10   Bankowski, Z., Howard-Jones, N., eds. *Human Experimentation and Medical Ethics*. Geneva: CIOMS, 1982.
11   Bankowski, Z., Howard-Jones, N., eds. *Biomedical Research Involving Animals: Proposed International Guiding Principles*. Geneva: CIOMS, 1984.
12   Bankowski, Z., Barzellato, J., Capron, A.M., eds. *Ethics and Human Values in Family Planning*. Geneva: CIOMS, 1989, 267.
13   Baral, V., Peterman, T.A., Berkelman, R., and Jaffe, H.W. "Kaposi's Sarcoma among Persons with AIDS: A Sexually Transmitted Infection." *Lancet* 1990, 1: 123-128.
14   Barry, M. "Ethical Considerations of Human Investigations in Developing Countries. The AIDS Dilemma." *New England Journal of Medicine* 1988, 319: 1083-1085.
15   Beauchamp, D.E. *The Health of the Republic: Epidemics, Medicine and Morality as Challenge to Democracy*. Philadelphia: Temple University Press, 1988, 67.
16   Black, D. "Health Care of the Elderly. Quality of Life and Aging." In: Bankowski, Z., Bryant, J.H., eds. *Health Policy, Ethics and Human Values*. Geneva: CIOMS, 1988, 137-142.
17   Blendon, R.J., Taylor, H. "A Health System that Needs Surgery." *New York*

Times May 9, 1989, A23.

18   Brahams, D. "Jehovah's Witness Transfused without Consent, A Canadian Case." *Lancet* 1989, 2: 1407-1408.

19   Bricker, E.M. "Industrial Marketing and Medical Ethics." *New England Journal of Medicine* 1989, 320: 1690-1692.

20   British Medical Association, *Euthanasia*. London: B.M.A., 1988.

21   Callahan, D. "Health Care of the Elderly. In: Bankowski, Z., Bryant, J.H. *Health Policy, Ethics and Human Values*. Geneva: CIOMS, 1988, 131-135.

22   Callahan, D. *Setting Limits: Medical Goals in an Aging Society*. New York: Simon and Shuster, 1987.

23   Capron, A.M. "Highlights of the Bangkok Conference." In: Bankowski, Z., Barzellato, J., Capron, A.M., eds. *Ethics and Human Values in Family Planning*. Geneva: CIOMS, 1989, 15-16.

24   Centers for Disease Control. Update: Acquired Immunodeficiency Syndrome-United States, 1989, *Journal of the American Medical Association* 1990, 263: 1191.

25   Chalmers, T.C. "Ethical Implications of Rejecting Patients for Clinical Trials." *Journal of the American Medical Association* 1990, 263: 865.

26   Chen, L.C., Cash, R.A. "A Decade after Alma Ata. Can Primary Health Care Lead to Health for All?" *New England Journal of Medicine* 1988, 319: 946-947.

27   Christakis, N.A. "The Ethical Design of an AIDS Vaccine Trial in Africa." *Hastings Center Report* 1988, 18: 31-37.

28   Colman, R.D. "The Ethics of General Practice and Advertising." *Journal of Medical Ethics* 1989, 15: 86-89, 93.

29   Concepcion, M.B. "Ethics and Human Values in Family Planning: Perspectives of Asia and Oceania." In: Bankowski, Z. Barzellato, J., Capron, A.M., eds. *Ethics and Human Values in Family Planning*. Geneva, CIOMS, 1989, 208-221.

30   Congress of the United States, Office of Technology Assessment. *Infertility: Medical and Social Choices*. Washington, D.C.: U.S. Government Printing Office, 1988.

31   Consultants of the Advisory Committee to the Director of the National Institutes of Health. *Report of the Human Fetal Tissue Transplant Panel*. Washington, D.C.: National Institutes of Health, 1988.

32   Council of Europe. Conference of European Health Ministers. 16-17 November 1987. *Organ Transplantation*. Strasbourg, 1987.

33   Cowan, D.H. "Gene Technology." *Journal of the American Medical Association* 1990, 263,16: 1571-1572.

34   Crisp, R. "Autonomy, Welfare and the Treatment of AIDS." *Journal of Medical Ethics* 1989, 15: 68-73.

35   Davies, N.E., Felder, L.H. "Applying Brakes to the Runaway American Health Care System." *Journal of the American Medical Association* 1990, 263: 73-76.

36   DeCraemer, W.A. "Cross-Cultural Perspective on Personhood." Milbank

Memorial Fund 1983, 61: 19-34.

37   deWachter, M.A.M. "Active Euthanasia in the Netherlands." *Journal of the American Medical Association* 1989, 262: 3316-3319.

38   Derby, J.M., Yonas, H., Crur, D., Latchaw, R.E. "Xenon-Enhanced Computed Tomography in Brain Death." *Archives of Neurology* 1987, 44: 551-556.

39   Dickens, B.M. "Morals and Markets in Transplantable Organs." *Transplantation Today* November 1989, 23-29.

40   Dickens, B.M. "Conference on Ethics, Justice and Commerce in Transplantation: A Global Issue." *International Digest of Health Legislation* 1990, 41: 179-182.

41   Dictor, M., Bendsoe, N., "Transmissible Agent or Kaposi's Sarcoma." *Lancet* 1990, 1: 797.

42   Eddy, D.M., Billings, J. "The Quality of Medical Evidence: Implications for Quality of Care." *Health Affairs* 7: 19-32.

43   Elias, S., Annas, G.J. *Reproductive Genetics and the Law.* Chicago: Year Book Medical Publishers, 1987.

44   "Embryo Research: The Standard Arguments." *Briefings in Medical Ethics*, 1990, 5: 1-3.

45   Engelhardt, H.T., Rie, M.A. "Morality for the Medical-Industrial Complex: A Code of Ethics for the Mass Marketing of Health Care." *New England Journal of Medicine* 1988, 319: 1086-1089.

46   "Exploring the Effectiveness of Healing." *Lancet* 1985, 2: 1177-1178.

47   "For Love or Money." Editorial. *Times* (of London), April 5, 1990, 15.

48   Fries, E.D. "Antihypertensive Agents." In: Kalow, W., Guedde, H.W., Agarwal, P., eds. *Ethnic Differences in Reactions to Drugs and Xenobiotics.* New York: Alan Liss, 1986, 312-322.

49   Fuchs, V.R. "The Rationing of Medical Care." *New England Journal of Medicine* 1984, 311: 1572-1573.

50   "Gene Therapy." Editorial. *Lancet* 1989, 1: 193-194.

51   "Gene Therapy in Man. Recommendations of European Medical Research Councils." *Lancet* 1988, 2: 1271-1272.

52   George, S. *A Fate Worse than Debt.* Uxbridge: Penguin, 1986.

53   Gillon, R. "Advertising and Medical Ethics." *Journal of Medical Ethics* 1989, 15: 59-60, 85.

54   Gillon, R. "Death." *Journal of Medical Ethics* 1990, 16:3-4.

55   Goodman, M.J., Goodman, E. "Medicalization and Its Discontents." *Social Sciences and Medicine* 1987, 25: 733-740.

56   Gorovitz, S. "Life, Suffering, Death, and Health Policies. The View of Secular Humanism." In: Bankowski, Z., Bryant, J.H., eds. *Health Policy, Ethics and Human Values.* Geneva: CIOMS, 1985, 45-46, 301-302.

57   Gorovitz, S. "Health Care in a Pluralistic System: Covering the Gaps." In: Bankowski, Z., Bryant, J.H., eds. *Health Policy, Ethics and Human Values.* Geneva: CIOMS, 1985, 233.

58   Greenfield, S. "The State of Outcome Research. Are We on Target?" *New*

England Journal of Medicine 1989, 320: 1142-1143.

59 "The Record Is One of Utter Despair." Editorial. *Guardian Newspaper* (United Kingdom), November 22, 1989, 2.

60 Hagenfeldt, K. "Ethics and Human Values in Family Planning. European and North American Perspectives." In: Bankowski, Z., Barzellato, J., Capron, A.M., eds. *Ethics and Human Values in Family Planning.* Geneva: CIOMS, 1989, 184-206.

61 Hathout, H. "Fundamental Values of Islam on Life, Suffering and Death- -Their Meaning for Medical Care and Social Justice." In: Bankowski, Z., Bryant, J.H., eds. *Health Policy, Ethics and Human Values.* Geneva: CIOMS, 304-307.

62 Hunter, S.F. "Active Euthanasia Violates Fundamental Principles." *Journal of the American Medical Association* 1989, 262: 3074.

63 Jabbari, D. "The Role of Law in Reproductive Medicine: A New Approach." *Journal of Medical Ethics* 1990, 16: 35-40.

64 Johnson, R., Siegler, M., Winslade, W.J. *Clinical Ethics* 3rd edition. New York: Macmillan, 1986.

65 Joseph, K.S. "The Matthew Effect in Health Development." *British Medical Journal* 1989, 298: 1497-1498.

66 Kalow, W. "Race and Therapeutic Drug Response." *New England Journal of Medicine* 1989, 320: 588-589.

67 Kassirer, J.P. "Our Stubborn Quest for Diagnostic Certainty." *New England Journal of Medicine* 1989, 320: 1489-1491.

68 Katzman, R. "Alzheimer's Disease." *New England Journal of Medicine* 1986, 314: 964-973.

69 "King Baudoin's Day Off." Editorial. *Times* (of London), April 5, 1990, 15.

70 Konetey-Ahulu, F.I.D. "AIDS in Africa: Misinformation and Disinformation." *Lancet* 1987, 2: 206-207.

71 Lace, T.J. "The Physicians Can Play a Positive Role in Euthanasia." *Journal of the American Medical Association* 1989, 262: 3075.

72 Lamb, D. "Brain Death Symposium. Commentary 1: Wanting It Both Ways." *Journal of Medical Ethics* 1990, 16: 8-9.

73 Laumn, R.D. *Mega Traumas: America at the Year 2000.* New York: Houghter Miffling Co., 1985.

74 Less Frequent Paps Called Sheer Idiocy." *Ob Gyn News*, December 1, 1982: 1.

75 Levin, D.M. "AIDS." *Journal of the American Medical Association* 1990, 263: 1715-1716.

76 Lillich, R.B. "Transplanting Organs from Living Donors: An International Regime or More Free Enterprise?" In: *Finnish Yearbook of International Law*, 1990. In press.

77 Luce, M. "Ethical Principles in Critical Care." *Journal of the American Medical Association* 1990, 263: 696-700.

78 G.D. Lundberg, "Countdown to Millenium. Balancing the Profession and Business of Medicine. Medicine's Rocking Horse." *Journal of the American*

Medical Association 1990, 263: 1.

79 Macklin, R. "Ethics and Human Values in Family Planning: Perspectives of Different Cultural and Religious Settings." In: Bankowski, Z., Barzellato, J., Capron, A.M., eds. *Ethics and Human Values in Family Planning.* Geneva: CIOMS, 1989, 68-85.

80 Madrazo, I., Leon, V., Torres, C. "Transplantation of Fetal Substantia Nigra and Adrenal Medulla to the Caudate Nucleus in Two Patients with Parkinson's Disease." *New England Journal of Medicine* 1988, 318: 51.

81 Manuel, C., Enel, P., Reviron, D., *et al.* "The Ethical Approach to AIDS: A Bibliographic Review." *Journal of Medical Ethics* 1990, 16: 14-27.

82 McGregor, M. "Technology and the Allocation of Resources." *New England Journal of Medicine* 1989, 320: 118-120.

83 McCormick, J.S. "Cervical Smears: A Questionable Practice?" *Lancet* 1989, 2: 207-209.

84 McKussick, V.A. "Mapping and Sequencing the Human Genome." *New England Journal of Medicine* 1989, 320: 910-915.

85 McLaren, A. "Keynote Address." In: Bankowski, Barzellato, J., Capron, A.M., eds. *Ethics and Human Values in Family Planning.* Geneva: CIOMS, 1989, 7-14.

86 Meyer-Lie, A. "The Political Abuse of Medicine." *Social Science and Medicine* 1987, 25: 645-648.

87 Miller, A.B. "Evaluation of Screening for Carcinoma or Cervix. *Modern Medicine in Canada* 1973, 28: 1067-1069.

88 Nevins, M.A. "New Jersey's Right-To-Die Cases: Round Three." *Annals of Internal Medicine* 1987, 107: 927-929.

89 Nolan, K. "Genug Ist Genug: A Fetus is not a Kidney." *Hastings Center Report* 1988, 18: 13-19.

90 Nowell-Smith, P. "Euthanasia and the Doctors--A Rejection of the B.M.A.'s Report." *Journal of Medical Ethics,* 1989, 15: 124-128.

91 Orientlicher, D. "Genetic Screening by Employers." *Journal of the American Medical Association* 1990, 263: 1005-1006.

92 Orr, A. "Legal AIDS: Implications of AIDS and HIV for British and American Law." *Journal of Medical Ethics* 1989, 15: 61-67.

93 Osuntokun, B.O. "Traditional Beliefs of Africa and Their Intersection with Modern Ideas and Beliefs: Implications for Health Policies." In: Bankowski, Z., Bryant, J.H., eds. *Health Policy, Ethics and Human Values.* Geneva: CIOMS, 1985, 274-286.

94 Osuntokun, B.O. "The Perspective of the Developing World Africa." In: Bankowski, Z., Bryant, J.H., eds. *Health Policy, Ethics and Human Values.* Geneva: CIOMS, 1988, 191-197.

95 Osuntokun, B.O., Ogunniyi, A.O., Lekwauwa, U.G., *et al.* "Epidemiology of Dementia in Nigerian Africans." In: *Proceedings: XIVth World Congress of Neurology.* New Delhi, India, October 22-27, 1989. Amsterdam, Excerpta Medica, 1990.

96 Pallis, C. "Brain Death Symposium. Commentary 2. Return to Elsinore." *Journal of Medical Ethics* 1990, 16: 10-13.

97 Paris, J.J., Reardon, F.E. "Dilemmas in Intensive Care Medicine: An Ethical and Legal Analysis." *Journal of Intensive Care Medicine* 1986, 1: 75-90.

98 Pellegrino, E.D. "Life, Death and Suffering from a Christian Perspective: Their Impact on Health Policy." In: Bankowski, Z., Bryant, J.H., eds. *Health Policy, Ethics and Human Values*. Geneva: CIOMS, 1985, 266-273.

99 Price, M. *Shattered Mirrors. Our Search for Identity and Community in the AIDS Era*. Cambridge: Harvard University Press, 1989.

100 *Proposed International Guidelines for Biomedical Research Involving Human Subjects*. Geneva: CIOMS, 1982.

101 Randall, J. "The Human Genome Project." *Lancet* 1989, 2: 1535-1536.

102 Ratanakul, P. "The Buddhist Concept of Life, Suffering and Death and Their Meaning for Health Policy," In: Bankowski, Z., Bryant, J.H., eds. *Health Policy, Ethics and Human Values*. Geneva: CIOMS, 1985, 286-295.

103 Reagan, M.D. "Health Care Rationing: What Does It Mean?" *New England Journal of Medicine* 1980, 319: 1149-1151.

104 Rees, G.J.G. "Cost-Effectiveness in Oncology." *Lancet* 1985, 2: 1405-1407.

105 Rix, B.A. "Danish Ethics Council Rejects Brain Death as the Criterion of Death." *Journal of Medical Ethics* 1990, 16: 5-7.

106 Roberts, C.J., Farrow, S.C., Charny, M.C. "How Much Can the NHS Afford to Spend to Save a Life or Avoid a Severe Disability?" *Lancet* 1985, 1: 89-91.

107 Rodwin, M.A. "Industrial Marketing and Medical Ethics." *New England Journal of Medicine* 1990, 322: 64.

108 Sabatier, R. "Blame and Counter-Blame in Blaming Others." London, Panos, 1988, 85-101.

109 Sagan, L.A., *The Health of Nations. True Causes of Sickness and Well-Being*. New York: Basic Books, 1987.

110 Salen, G., Tint, G.S. "TIMI II and the Role of Angioplasty in Acute Myocardial Infarction." *New England Journal of Medicine* 1989, 320: 663-666.

111 Sell, R., Kunitz, S. "The Debt Crisis and the End of an Era in Mortality Decline," *Studies in Comparative International Development* 1987.

112 Serwadda, D., Katongole-Mbidde, E. "AIDS in Africa: Problems for Research and Researchers." *Lancet* 1990, 1: 842-843.

113 Sheldon, M. "Truth-Telling in Medicine." *Journal of the American Medical Association* 1982, 247: 651-654.

114 Skoda, R.C., Gonzalez, F.J., Demierre, A., Mayer, H.A., "Two Mutant Alleles of the Human Cytochrome P-450 dbl Gene (P450C21) Associated with Genetically Deficient Metabolism of Debrisoquine and Other Drugs." *Proceedings of the National Academy of Science, USA* 1988, 85: S240-S243.

115 Skolnick, A. "Gene Replacement Therapy for Hereditary Emphysema?" *Journal of the American Medical Association* 1989, 262: 2489.

116 Stanley, J.M. "The Appleton Consensus: Suggested International Guidelines for Decisions to Forego Medical Treatment." *Journal of Medical Ethics*

1989, 15: 129-136.

117 Steinberg, A. "Religious Values of Judaism about Life, Sufferings and Death. The Message for Policymakers." In: Bankowski, Z., Bryant, J.H. *Health Policy, Ethics and Human Values*. Geneva: CIOMS, 1985, 262-265.

118 Stjernswald, J. "Plotting a New Course for Cervical Cancer Screening in Developing Countries." *World Health Forum* 1987, 8: 42-45.

119 Summerfield, D. "Western Economies and Third World Health." *Lancet* 1989, 2: 551-552.

120 Swenson, S. "Depo-Provera: Loopholes and Double Standards." *Hastings Center Report* 1987, 17: 3.

121 Townsend, P., Davidson, N. *Inequalities in Health*. Hammondsworth: Penguin, 1982.

122 Truog, R.D., Fletcher, J.C. "Anencephalic Newborns: Can Organs be Transplanted Before Brain Death?" *New England Journal of Medicine* 1989, 321: 388-391; and 1990, 322: 333.

123 van der Werff, A. "Health Policy, Ethics and Organ Transplantation." In: Bankowski, Z., Bryant, J.H., eds. *Health Policy, Ethics and Human Values*. Geneva: CIOMS, 1985, 206-216.

124 Villard, L., Murphy, M., Vessey, M.P., "Cervical Cancer Deaths in Young Women." *Lancet* 1989, 1: 377.

125 Wagner, M.G., St. Clair, P.A., "Are In-Vitro Fertilization and Embryo Transfer of Benefit to All?" *Lancet* 1989, 2: 1027-1029.

126 Walkie, F.L., Eisdorfer, C., Morgan, R., Loewenstein, D.A., Szapocznik, J. "Cognition in Early Human Immunodeficiency Virus Infection." *Archives of Neurology* 1990, 47: 433-440.

127 Walters, L. "The Ethics of Human Gene Therapy." *Nature* 1986, 320: 225-227.

128 Wanzer, S.H., Federman, D.D., Adelstein, J., *et al*. "The Physician's Responsibility Towards Hopelessly Ill Patients." *New England Journal of Medicine* 1989, 320: 844-849.

129 Wasi, P. "Scientific and Public Policy Problems of Thalassaemia in Thailand." In: Bankowski, Z., Bryant, J.H. *Health Policy, Ethics and Human Values*. Geneva: CIOMS, 1985, 146-153.

130 "Zimbabwe Faces Dictatorship." Editorial. Winnipeg Free Press. April 9, 1990, 8.

131 *World Bank Debt Tables* 1987-88, 2.

132 World Health Assembly, Geneva, Resolution WAA, 425.

133 World Health Organization, Global Programme on AIDS. *Report of the Consultation on the Neuropsychiatric Aspects of HIV Infection*. Geneva: WHO, March 14-17, 1988.

134 World Health Organization, Global Programme on AIDS. *Neuropsychiatric Aspects of HIV-1 Infection: A Review of the Evidence*. Report of the Consultation held in Geneva. Geneva: WHO, January 11-13, 1990.

135 Zhou, H.H., Koshakji, R.P., Silberstein, D.J., Wilkinson, G.P., Wood, A.J.J.

"Racial Differences in Drug Response: Altered Sensitivity to and Clearance of Propranolol in Men of Chinese Descent as Compared with American Whites." *New England Journal of Medicine* 1989, 320: 565-570.

136 Zwi, A.B. "The Political Abuse of Medicine and the Challenge of Opposing It." *Social Science and Medicine* 1987, 25: 649-657.

11

Conflict and Harmony in Japanese Medicine: A Challenge to Traditional Culture in Neonatal Care

Rihito Kimura

SOCIO-HISTORICAL BACKGROUND OF JAPANESE MEDICINE

In 1984 in Japan, the 1000th anniversary of the publication of *Ishimpo* was celebrated. This is the oldest extant book of medicine consisting of thirty volumes edited and written from Chinese and Japanese medical resources by Yasuyori Tanba in 984.[13,15]

While reading the Ansei edition (1859) of this book, kept in the National Library of Congress, Washington, DC, I was very much impressed with the unique Japanese expression in Chinese characters of *taijisokuin* relating to the practice of healing.[13] The word *taiji* (the great mercy of Buddha) was taken from Buddhist Scripture and the other part of the word *sokuin* (sympathy, benevolence) was taken from Confucian books such as the *Analects*. According to my analysis in reading this book, it is clear that there is a long tradition in Japanese medical practice which appeals to the healing power of traditional Shinto gods, as well as to Buddhist and Confucian teaching.

In particular, the Confucian notion of *sokuin*, which is usually regarded as the same notion as *jin*, has been one of the most important ethical elements in the long tradition of teaching Confucianism and medical theory. Practice was well developed in the framework of the Confucian ethos based on the Confucian understanding of nature, human life, and disease. In fact, medicine in the Japanese tradition is always referred to as the *art of jin* or *jinjyutsu*.[3,14]

Even though Western medicine has had some impact since the sixteenth century, there was no radical change in the medical system and education until the middle of the nineteenth century. Total reorientation of modern medical science occurred after the official opening of Japan to the West in 1868, when the

German influence in the field of medicine became dominant.[7] However, the Japanese mentality, nurtured in the Confucian ethos which emphasizes respect for law, order, authority, and social status, did not change even after the rapid modernization of Japanese society brought about by the adoption of Western science and technology.

Reflecting these social values in human relationships, physicians in Japan have, until recently, continued their typically paternalistic and authoritative behavior towards patients and their family members. Parents have also felt comfortable yielding authority to prestigious physicians. In Japanese society, which is structured on traditional family values, each person is expected to behave in a modest non-assertive way with full sensitivity to "harmony" in relationships with other people, particularly with professionals such as physicians, government officers, and superiors in the work place. Avoiding confrontation in human relationships by not pointing out clear differences in philosophy, opinion, and policy, Japanese have the tendency to be the same in a family or organization. Japanese society is quite a contrast to Western society which encourages people to be "unique." "Different" means "strange" in Japanese, and this strangeness has had a negative implication in Japanese culture. However, the Japanese have had an enormous interest in this "strangeness" and strive to "Japanize" strange things and thoughts from overseas. In this light, Western medicine, when it was first introduced, was regarded as particularly strange for many Japanese, and yet was eagerly adopted.

DECISIONMAKERS: WHO AND WHY?

In the context of the uniquely formed Japanese social setting, physicians, patients, and family members are now facing various types of complicated bioethical problems relating to medical services, particularly neonatal care. Because of the rapid development in medical science and technology in setting up NICUs (neonatal intensive care units), some newborns who would have died now survive. However, they might possibly suffer later from such conditions as chronic cardiopulmonary disease, short bowel syndrome, or various brain damage manifestations and/or severe handicaps as a result of various congenital malformations.

Physicians have the following attitude: "No one can decide whether or not someone is worth saving. A newborn baby with a devastating disorder cannot make a decision one way or another. If we physicians cannot make such a decision, who can?" This shows that the process of decisionmaking is grounded in a sense of professional responsibility based on a framework of traditional Japanese paternalistic approaches. More and more, Japanese patients and their families are questioning this kind of attitude. However, quite a number of physicians in Japan are still holding on to this paternalistic view in the decisionmaking process as something quite natural and a part of professional medical discretion. Physicians usually defend this attitude by asking: Can parents in a traumatic situation resulting from the birth of a handicapped child understand what faces them? Can they exercise truly informed consent for treatment or for withholding treatment? Behind these questions raised by conscientious, experienced physicians, there is the premise that, for the benefit of the patient, it is acceptable not to tell the whole truth to the patient, parents, and family members.[2]

It might also be the case that, even if the doctor were to tell the whole truth to the patient, the decision of the family regarding the life or death of the baby would still be influenced by the physician. A physician might limit or manipulate disclosure of information relating to the diagnosis and prognosis of the patient. Thus, even in the face of a growing patients' rights movement, many Japanese physicians still believe that "medical decisionmaking" should be borne primarily by attending physicians who generally make little effort to reflect on medical decisions or on the ethical and value decisionmaking of the patient and family.[10]

In spite of the paternalistic tendency in Japanese medical care, it is also common to have some sort of "sharing process" involved when making medical decisions. In this sense, the Japanese type of professional paternalism is not always a dictatorial type of relationship, but, rather, involves a sense of shared group responsibility. This sense of group responsibility makes it easy for Japanese to work together, whether it is in a large industrial organization, or in the process of reaching a decision between parents and physicians regarding a neonatal case.[11]

In neonatal care, no definitive guidelines have been reached, but there is a consensus in such cases as anencephaly, hydroanencephaly, and trisomy 18 that the baby should be allowed to die. The following case regarding the care of a handicapped newborn in Japan is reported by Dr. Masamichi Sakanoue, Professor of Pediatrics and neonatology at Kitasato University Medical School:

> A male infant was born after 26 weeks of gestation at a weight of about 800 grams. Because of an immature lung, he was mechanically ventilated. During early intensive care, he developed congestive heart failure due to patent ductus arteriosus which was subsequently ligated surgically. Because of the irreversible damage to the lung, the baby could not be weaned off the ventilator. This condition is categorized as bronchopulmonary dysplasia. It was impossible to give milk because of frequent gastric residual and persistent paralytic ileus. Nutritional elements were administered intravenously to the baby, but it was inadequate for proper growth. In this situation, he remained relatively stable for six months on mechanical ventilation. At six months, his weight was only 1200 grams. At that time no blood vessels for giving nutrition could be found and there was very little hope that he would ever breathe and nurse by himself. Finally he developed systematic infection and his condition gradually deteriorated. Further medical treatment was given up by the medical team, and he was allowed to die.

Professor Sakanoue explained that he shared almost all of the decisionmaking process with the parents, though not the full medical details when decisions were purely professional. He felt it was unwise to tell every detail to the parents, mentioning clearly that he believes it is very cruel for physicians to ask parents make the final decision regarding their baby's fate.

In this type of decisionmaking process, the role of nurses is very important. Typically, the neonatal team consisting of physicians, nurses, and social workers maintains close communication by means of daily medical conferences.

In this sharing process, care of the babies becomes a holistic approach in which cooperation among members of the medical team is encouraged. Figure 1 shows the important role of nurses in forming this positive shared approach to the care of newborns.

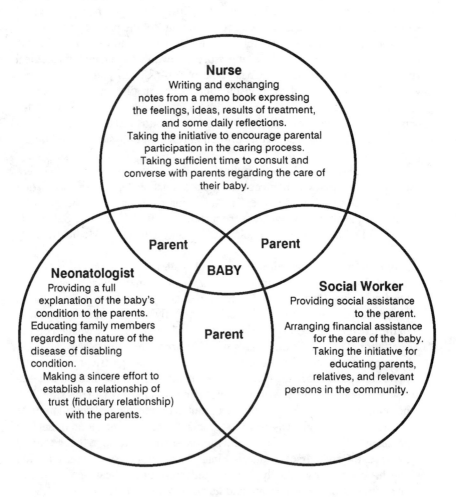

Figure 1. Roles in the Caring Process of Handicapped Newborns

One of the unique practices of Japanese nurses in the area of neonatal care is their relationship with the parents of a newly born handicapped child. As shown in the nurse's role on the chart, they do not share only the problem and process of medical treatment. They also exchange their feelings and discuss the baby's situation with the parents by writing memos, as these expressions are sometimes very delicate and difficult to express in oral communication. The initiative for this note-writing is usually taken by nurses, and the contents of several comments in the notebook are read by the physician on the team who also will write some comments. Thus physicians, nurses, and parents of the baby, as well as family members, all contribute to the care of the newborns. Table 1 shows this cooperative support system focusing on the newly born handicapped child in the Japanese hospital setting.

Table 1
Cooperation in the Support System for Care of Handicapped Newborns

Medical Team	Social and Institutional Support System
Gynecologist	Health/medical benefits
Pediatrician/Neonatologist	Insurance (state, local, government, private)
Anesthesiologist	Acceptance of the baby in the family support system
Neurosurgeon	
Plastic Surgeon	Arrangement of the care network through a local health center (*Hokenjyo*) by visiting public health nurses
Physical Therapist	
Orthopedist	Legal protection of the baby's right to life
General Practitioner (Family Physician)	Psychological support by social workers
Nurse/Public Health Nurse (*Hokenfu*)	
Genetic Counselor	

THE NETWORK OF NEONATAL CARE

Neonatal care could not be effective if approached only through health care oriented to the patient alone. Thus, concerned neonatologists have proposed that it is necessary to establish a national neonatal network system with regional neonatal care centers all over Japan.[8] It is also very important that these kinds of regional centers for the care of neonates be specialized in regard to particular medical conditions and that they be located conveniently. The facilities should be of adequate size and be able to meet varying local needs. There should be a good support system linking these centers to the general clinic or hospital which, ideally, would have close contact with practicing physicians in the local communities.

Regional neonatal care centers with local orientations would particularly benefit from having various resources in one place, so that caring activities and their management would be more effectively administered by the well-qualified specialists at the centers. As care for neonates sometimes demands very expensive medical engineering and electronic equipment, technologists responsible for this would be part of the team. Regional networking of these centers would give tremendously effective services to local communities, making available systematically-monitored screening for medical problems or possible prematurity.[16]

There have already been some regional efforts to apply a systematic approach to solve locally unique problems relating to the case of newborns. For example, Kagawa Prefecture in Shikoku (one of the main islands of Japan), was known for many years as having a high mortality rate among newborns. However, this changed very drastically after the systematic regional network for neonatal care was adopted. Today, Kagawa Prefecture has one of the lowest infant mortality rates in Japan. Similarly, in Kanagawa Prefecture near Tokyo, there has been an effective network for neonatal care because of the full cooperation between pediatricians and gynecologists in public and private medical institutions. Also in Kanagawa Prefecture, detailed network-planning for an "emergency care system" for potentially high risk mothers and infants is under way.[9]

As a result of these positive experiences in the networking of neonatal care in several regions and communities, a proposal was made for establishment of neonatal care centers as a part of a national system. To be most effective while also respecting the rights of the patient and family, I think there should be some basic guidelines for comprehensive care of newborns in these regional neonatal centers. Some of the tasks to be developed under such guidelines would be as follows:

● Develop a systematic medical and social team approach (see Figure 1 and Table 1).
● Insure the effective use of ME equipment and NICUs.
● Organize educational and training programs for specialists in neonatal care. These include physicians, nurses, and social workers. Other related persons including parents, local public officials, and the lay public should also

receive some relevant form of education.
- Promote and develop the national neonatal network information system for the care of the newborns. This would be a multidisciplinary assistance and communication system using computer technology.
- Exchange information regarding neonatal care and emergency action when necessary for hospitalization, consultation in transfer cases, etc.
- Establish an effective local network for neonatal care in local and regional communities.

Overall, the neonatal care system has received enormous attention during the past several years, particularly after the epoch-making birth of quintuplets in Japan in 1976. Thus, even in the traditional framework of paternalistic Japanese medicine, we are now able to recognize several changes in attitude towards medical care among both medical professionals and patients. One important progressive practice resulting from these changes is the sharing of decisionmaking which we have observed in neonatal care units. It also appears that the younger Japanese generation has a tendency to prefer the truth concerning the diagnosis and prognosis of any disease, particularly in the case of cancer.

CONCLUDING REMARKS

As I have shown in the example of the nurse's unique initiative in neonatal care, a sense of sharing is one of the important Japanese principles honored in bioethical decisionmaking. This sharing of *kyokan* (feeling of togetherness) as *ningen* (human person in a relational context) could be interpreted as part of our Japanese Buddhist tradition.[12] The principle of autonomy, usually referred to as one of the important bioethical principles in the Western social context, might not apply effectively within the Japanese cultural tradition. This is because Japanese culture, nurtured in Buddhist teaching, has developed the idea that the egoistic self should be completely suppressed. To be autonomous and independent as an individual has been regarded as an egocentric idea, one which does not address the need for people to be dependent on each other in the family, social, economic, and political community. This unique understanding of the Japanese character analyzed by Dr. Takeo Doi in his book, *The Anatomy of Dependence*,[12] further explains the background of the "sharing principle" in the Japanese bioethics which I have been advocating.[4]

Thus, a Japanese perspective of neonatal care can be summarized by saying that the ancient and well-rooted Japanese principle of sharing is taken seriously in the relationship between parents and the neonatal care providers in local and regional communities, as well as in the national setting.[1] As a result, the long-standing paternalistic tradition within the Japanese medical community is partially overcome.

NOTES

1   Doi, T. "The Anatomy of Dependence (Amae no Kozo)." New York, 1973.
2   Ishida, T. "Values, Norms and Education." *Japanese Society* 1971, 37-48; see also: Jacobson, N.P. *The Japan Way*. Tokyo, 1977, 24-37.
3   Kaibara, E. *Yojokun*. Edo (Tokyo), 1713. English translation by Masao Kunihiro under the title *YOJOKUN--Japanese Secret to Good Health*, Tokyo, 1974, 119.
4   Kimura, R. "Bioethical Thought in Asia--The Internationalization of the Notion of Jin (Iwa Jinjyutsu no Kokusaika). In: Byoin *The Japanese Journal of Hospital*, 1982, 41, no.7:60-61.
5   Kimura, R. "Bioethics as 'Sharing Principle'--Sharing of Information, Sharing of Decisions and Sharing of Strategy in Byoin." *Japanese Journal of Hospital* 1982, 41, no.9:52-53.
6   Kimura, R. Steslicke, W.E. "Medical Technology for the Elderly in Japan." *International Journal of Technology Assessment in Health Care* 1985, 1, no.1:37. See note 7. Using the same approach as that applied in geriatric technology, a kind of 'soft wear' service and care would be applied to neonatal care when faced with the need for neonatal technology.
7   Oshima, T. "The Japanese-German System of Medical Education, History of Medical Education." Proceedings of the 6th International Symposium on the Comparative History of Medicine--East and West. Tokyo, 1983.
8   Nakane, C. "*Tate* Shakai no Rikigaku." (The Dynamics of Vertical Society). Tokyo, 1978, 126-129.
9   Nishida, H. "NICU o Megette (On NICU)." In: *Medical Way*, 1985, 2, no.2:27.
10   Sakanoue, M. "Contemporary Medical Service and Ethics in Medicine." *Journal of Freedom and Justice* (Jiyu to Seigi), 1983, 34, no.7:7-8 and Masamichi S., *et al.* "The Progress of Medicine and Bioethics." In: *Life Sciences and Religion II*. Tokyo, 1982, 163-164.
11   Sakanoue, M., Nishida, H. "Case Studies on the Decision-Making Process for Newborn Babies of Pruneberry Syndrome and 18 Trisomy." *Shoinka Shinryo (The Japanese Journal of Pediatric Therapeutics)*, 1981, 44:8.
12   Sukawa, Y. "Sentenijo no Hasseiyobo to Boshihoken (The Protection of Hereditary Abnormality and Health of Mothers and Children)." 1983, 68-80.
13   Tanba, Y. *Inshinpo*, 984. See also: *Ishimpo 1000 nen no Ayumi*. Tokyo: Society for the Commemoration of the One Thousandth Anniversary of the "Ishimpo" (Drawing of Japanese Medicine-Ishimpo-), 1984, English translation was partially done by Akira Ishihara and H.S. Levy under the title *The Tao of Sex*. An annotated translation of the 28th section of the essence of medical prescription-Ishimpo, 1969, Yokohama, Japan.
14   E. Kaibara says in 1713 in *Yojokun* that "I wa Jinjyutsu nari" which means, "The medicine is an art of jin" (humanitarian art). On page 120 Kaibara says that anyone who aspires to become a doctor should become well-versed in the Confucian classics.

The most well-read recent edition of *Yojokun* is the Iwanami edition. (Iwanami-Bunko) published in 1961. (22nd printing of this edition in 1980).

Around 80 percent of contemporary Japanese physicians concur that this idea of Jinjyutsu, based on the Confucian notion, is a correct understanding of medical practice. (Based on a survey done by the *Nikkei Medical Journal*, May and June issues, 1975).

15   The greater Washington, DC area has very good documentation resource facilities for the research of Japanese medical ethics. Both the National Library of Congress and the National Library of Medicine have kept many valuable Japanese medical classics since the 18th century. The US National Record Center at Suitland, Maryland has kept all the documents related to Public Health Administration on under the GHQ's General Sams. The most recent declassified document shows the secret deal of the United States Medical Corps with Japanese war criminals who underwent human experimentation in Manchuria (Northern China) during the war. See Gomer, R., Powell, J.W., and Roling, B.V.A. "Japan's Biological Weapons 1930-1945," *Bulletin of the Atomic Scientists*, 1981, 37, no.8.

16   Both Figure 1 and Table 1 are the author's modifications of a chart developed originally by Dr. Masamichi Sakanoue. These were based on his clinical practice in the comprehensive team approach at the pediatric/neonatal care department of Kitasato University Hospital, Kanagawa, Japan. Also see Masamichi Sakanoue, Gendai Iryo no Jirenma (The dilemma of contemporary medicine) in *Pathema Quarterly*, 1982, 3.

12

Medical Ethics and Chinese Culture

Ren-Zong Qiu

INTRODUCTION

This paper consists of three sections. In the first section, I sketch the development of Chinese medical ethics with a focus on the contemporary stage of this development. The second section is devoted to the characteristics of Chinese contemporary medical ethics in comparison with its Western counterpart. In the third section, I attempt to provide an explanation of these characteristics in terms of Chinese culture and to highlight the influence of Chinese culture on medical ethics.

SECTION ONE

Chinese medicine has a history of at least two thousand years. The first explicit literature on medical ethics did not appear until the seventh century when a physician named Sun Simiao wrote a famous treatise titled "On the Absolute Sincerity of Great Physicians" in his work *The Important Prescriptions Worth a Thousand Pieces of Gold.*[16] In this treatise, later called the Chinese Hippocratic Oath, Sun Simiao requires the physician to develop first a sense of compassion and piety, and then to make a commitment to try to save every living creature, to treat every patient on equal grounds, and to avoid seeking wealth because of his expertise.

Traditional Chinese medical ethics is the application of Confucianism in the field of medical care. Confucian ethics is a form of virtue ethics with a strong deontological basis. Its focus has been on the virtues that a moral agent should have and the ways they can be acquired. The starting point of this morality is the cultivation of one's character by becoming a person with compassion. All the requisites which a physician should meet, and all the maxims that he or she should follow without regard to consequences, are heavenly principles.

In premodern China, medical ethical issues were addressed only in the preface of medical texts. All maxims, exhortations, admonitions, and warnings were personal advice or suggestions of well-known and prestigious physicians of that time. These guidelines were based on the personal experience of noted physicians, but were not professional codes in any sense. There have never been medical professional organizations in traditional China, so codes would not have any binding power on physicians.[10] Only on January 1, 1937, was "The Creed of Doctors" published by the Chinese Association of Doctors as the motto of modern medical practitioners in China.[18]

In 1949, after the founding of the People's Republic of China, the government cancelled the licensing system. Even though mistaken medical judgments were made after this time, the courts and lawyers were not allowed to become involved. Social control of medical practice relied mainly on regulations of health administrations and ideological education by the Communist Party Committee of Hospitals. Medical personnel were required to read Mao's article titled "In Memory of Comrade Norman Bethune" and to generate criticism and self-criticism according to Mao's teachings before and during the notorious Cultural Revolution.

Medical ethics has become one of the most flourishing disciplines in the People's Republic of China during the last decade. The current stage of Chinese medical ethics began with a conference on the philosophy of medicine which was held in Canton in December of 1979. At the plenary session of this conference a report titled "Philosophical Issues of Medicine in the 1970s" was made, part of which was devoted to medical ethics.[11] After this conference the discussion of medical ethics focussed on two issues: the concept of death and euthanasia, and the delivery of medical care without discrimination.[11] Before the publicity of two legal cases, one on active euthanasia, the other on artificial insemination by donor (AID),[15] the discussion was circumscribed by academic and professional circles. These circles were comprised of physicians, philosophers, and health care administrators who were publishing in specialized journals and attending conferences or colloquia on philosophy of medicine or medical ethics.

After the publicity on the cases, medical ethics drew attention from lawyers, journalists, policymakers, legislators, and the public. For example, after broadcasting divergent opinions about the first legal case on active euthanasia in a dialogue aired on a popular program called "Half Hour at Noon,"[10] Central People's Broadcasting Station received more than a thousand letters from its audience all over China. Of them, 85 percent favored some form of euthanasia, while 15 percent--including a school girl in the fifth grade of a primary school--were against any form of euthanasia. The widow of the late Premier Zhou Enlai, Mrs. Deng Yinchao, took the time to write a letter to the station to support the discussion. She said: "A couple of years ago, I wrote a living will to the effect that when I become terminally ill and medicine is no longer useful, the effort to save my life must not be made."

In January of 1989, another discussion on euthanasia was aired by the Central People's Broadcasting Station on a program called "English Service." The First National Conference on Social, Ethical, and Legal issues relating to euthanasia was held in Shanghai in June of 1988 with an attendance of 112 physicians, medical scientists, nurses, philosophers, lawyers, and health care administrators.

Euthanasia

During this decade, one of the primary medical ethical issues to be addressed is euthanasia. There are two Chinese translations of the English word "euthanasia": *anlesi* which means peaceful and happy dying, and *wutongzhisi* which means painless killing. The first is more widely accepted.

On almost every point there has been dissent among physicians, philosophers, lawyers, and the public. At the Shanghai conference on euthanasia, only one thing was agreed on unanimously by all participants: the suggestion that the criterion for death of the person be brain death. The other suggestion was that society ought to accept the right of a terminally ill patient to choose his or her way of dying and should encourage the practice of writing a living will. These recommendations were accepted by all but two participants.[7]

However, there seems to be common assent that the following four kinds of patients fall within the category of those for whom euthanasia may be considered: the comatose, the terminally ill, seriously defective newborns, and very low birth weight infants. If the criterion of brain death is accepted and the irreversibly comatose can be defined as dead, they should not be excluded from the category.[13]

Can euthanasia be identified as a special modality of death differentiated from natural death, accidental death, suicide, murder, and manslaughter? At the Shanghai conference, some participants characterized it in the following way:

> Under the condition of expressing her or his will orally or written, previously or presently, patients who are terminally ill and not incompetent (may reasonably request euthanasia). If no living will is left, the withholding or withdrawal of useless, painful, or burdensome treatment or active measures to end his or her life painlessly may be taken out of compassion and a desire to be of assistance. (Such an act) is done out of respect for his or her dignity and right to choose a way of dying. If the person is incompetent, these procedures may not be done against his or her will.[7]

It was argued that this characterization can be applied to the seriously defective newborn and very low birth weight infant with some modification. The problem in the case of euthanasia as characterized above is: What is the cause of death? Is it the action of withholding or withdrawing treatment, the action of ending life, or the disease process? Another problem is: How can the motive of this action be classified? Was it done from compassion or from some selfish intention?

Is euthanasia ethically justifiable? Most Chinese ethicists argue that the principles of beneficence, autonomy, and justice can be applied to justify euthanasia in certain circumstances. But behind the agreement there is a discrepancy in the argument. The holistic argument is that which emphasizes the benefit euthanasia may bring to the whole society. The argument from individualism is that we should respect the right of the terminally ill to choose a way of dying that is in his or her best interests. If a terminally ill patient prefers to live as long as possible no matter how painful the life will be, and there is no financial problem to prevent access to the needed medical care, we should respect her or his choice.

There have been cases in which patients committed suicide by hanging themselves, or have cut an artery with a knife, or have jumped from a window after their request to withdraw treatment was refused. Physicians felt themselves to be in an embarrassing dilemma when faced with such cases. Euthanasia can help us to avoid these tragic outcomes. In the case of seriously defective newborns and very low birth weight infants, euthanasia is intended to prevent an existence filled with suffering, at least in the current circumstances of China. It can be seen in letters from radio and television audiences who respond favorably to the idea of euthanasia. One elderly person wrote: "I don't want to die in a painful way." Another person who had the experience of caring for a terminally ill relative wrote: "I have no heart to see my kin dying in such a way."

On the other hand, the main objections brought forth against euthanasia are:

Psychological   When people are close to death, they often have a stronger will to continue life.

Ethical   The heavenly principle of medical ethics prohibits a physician from doing anything which might bring the patient closer to death.

Social   Any form of euthanasia can be misused as a disguise for murder.

Medical   Euthanasia will hinder the development of medicine.

Does euthanasia violate existing Chinese law? Most Chinese lawyers give a positive answer. Euthanasia violates the existing Chinese marital law, criminal law, and civil law. In the official explanation of criminal law, there are two factors which are very important in judging if an action constitutes a murder: one is motive--whether or not the agent intends the death of the innocent victim; the other is effect--whether the action is the cause of the victim's death. In the case of euthanasia, the motive of the agent and the effect of the intervening action are the same as in the case of murder. However, some have suggested that it is possible to change the current explanation by applying the principle of double effect.[7]

Is euthanasia acceptable to the Chinese public? Surveys show that the percentage of respondents favoring active euthanasia as well as passive euthanasia is higher than we expected. In a survey which my colleagues and I made in 1985,[13] four actual cases were described: a newborn with serious heart disease (cardianastorophe, angioplany, hypoplastic left heart, ventricular septal defect, auricular septal defect); a one-month-old female baby with microencephaly; an irreversibly comatose patient; and a dying cancer patient with intractable pain. The percentage favoring euthanasia was 14.7 percent, 62.4 percent, 37.1 percent, and 39.4 percent, respectively. In the first case, 42.9 percent of the respondents favored the parents as final decisionmakers, whereas 33.5 percent favored a committee, and only 17.1 percent thought that the physician should make the decision alone. In the second case, 58.5 percent of the respondents held the view that even though a one-month-old baby is a person, it is permissible to take his or her life if that quality of life is very low. Another survey showed that 37.09 percent of respondents favored euthanasia and 46.02 percent thought that it should be done by specialized workers. In this survey, 54.97 percent thought that the decision should be made by consultation between physician and family, 26.82 percent favored the patient as decisionmaker, and 8.94 percent favored the physician. One interesting finding was that attitudes towards euthanasia reflect professional, educational, and age differences. Respondents who were medical personnel or engaged in other intellectual pursuits, the well-educated, and young people held a more favorable attitude toward euthanasia.[3]

These surveys show that more and more Chinese medical personnel and laypersons take quality of life into account when considering euthanasia. The respondents reflected a balance of different values. Both the principle of respect for the sanctity of life embodied in the practice of making every effort to prolong life no matter what the cost and the paternalism embodied in the practice of decisionmaking by the physician without informed consent seem to be weakened. A story of a peasant who rescued a diseased pig was published on the first page of *People's Daily* and praised as a model of moral action. Another similar story was that of a train which made an unscheduled stop at a station so that an ill passenger could be treated. We can see that a change in the focus of morality has taken place since the Cultural Revolution.

Reproductive Technology

Reproductive technology as it is now practiced or being developed through research in China includes prenatal sex selection, artificial insemination by husband (AIH), artificial insemination by donor (AID), and in vitro fertilization (IVF). AIH seems not to have raised any ethical issues. Procedures such as IVF and organ transplantation, which require advanced technology to implement, are limited by Chinese policy to development in a few centers.

The application and development of reproductive technology benefits infertile couples. Among newly married couples, the rate of infertility is approximately 5 to 10 percent.[20] Where the reproductive technology has not been available, people have resorted to other means such as the practice of a "borrowed wife" to solve their problems. In some villages, infertile couples have agreed to pay a "borrowed wife" and her husband payments of 10,000 yuan (about US $2000) for a girl and 20,000 yuan (about US $4000) for a boy. This practice can be called "surrogate motherhood by natural insemination."

In China, AIH and AID are now widely practiced. Sperm banks have been set up in eleven provinces.[7] In Beijing and Changsha, "test tube babies" have been born after conception by IVF, and people are currently considering surrogate motherhood.

While doctors have been working out the technical problems in reproductive technology, the related social, ethical, and legal issues have gained increasing public interest. After sex identification by amniocentesis, 90 percent of female fetuses were aborted. In 1986, the male to female ratio of infants was 108.4:100. Now it is about 112:100[5] which may be due mainly to what is termed "postnatal selection," that is, female infanticide (a crime under existing laws). Prenatal sex selection is also a factor. The Ministry of Health currently prohibits the practice of prenatal sex selection.[8]

Except in a few centers in larger cities, there has been no regulation of IVF. Those who practice AID do not apply any criteria for selection of either donors or recipients: there are no special procedures required, no application forms in which the success of the procedure or the condition of the child could be confirmed, no records, no follow-up studies, and so on. Even private doctors at the community level practice AID using as a donor, perhaps, the shoemaker who happens to live near the gate. Fees are charged, so doctors engaging in this practice receive a considerable amount of money from infertile patients.

The legal status of AID children is not guaranteed. There was a case in Shanghai[8] which illustrated the conflict between traditional values and modern technology. In this case, the AID child was not given legal status and was not accepted by the extended family. This was due to the fact that their traditional values did not allow for one who does not come from the blood lineage of the husband's family to be recognized as part of that family.

Family Planning

Family planning and the policy of "one couple, one child" is the most thorny problem in China. In order to cope with overpopulation, the Chinese must do something to control this difficulty. The goal of the public on this matter is to make sure that the Chinese population does not exceed 1.2 billion by the year

2000. But it is not so easy to achieve such a goal because a slowing of population growth is in conflict with the government's new economic policy, with Chinese traditional values, and with the wishes of a great number of peasants. The results of an unpublished survey made by the Chinese Society for Sociology in 1979 shows that a considerable percentage of city inhabitants (19.44-30.95 percent) and the majority of peasants (51.34-79.53 percent) want to have two or more children. The issues involved are:

1. Is it ethically justifiable for a government to limit the right of its citizens to reproduce? I think that, in principle, I agree with Professor H. Tristam Engelhardt on this question. He argues: "Reproduction, unlike sexual intercourse, concerns more than the consenting individuals providing gametes. The production of a new person involves not only obligations of parents towards children, but also their duties towards society and others who may become financially obliged to protect and nurture the new individual."[21]

2. Although the limitation may be justifiable in principle, what should be done when the policy runs counter to the wishes of many people? Whenever this occurs, either the use of coercion is necessary to achieve compliance or the policy becomes unenforceable. There is little difficulty in big cities, where most inhabitants favor having one child, but in some rural areas either the rate of growth of population is beyond the limit of the government, or, in certain so-called advanced areas of family planning, there is some form of coercion.

3. How much emphasis should be focussed on abortion? The government claims that the primary emphasis in population control policy is on contraception, not abortion. But in rural areas, contraception has been unsuccessful and so the peasants resort to abortion. From 1971 to 1983 the number of abortions totalled 92 million. Since 1983, the figure has not been available.

4. Although, generally speaking, abortion is not considered to be an issue in China, what should be done about the risks and problems posed to all concerned? Many women in rural areas have undergone abortion so many times that officials responsible for maternal care worry about their health. In addition, since there is no problem in using the tissues or organs of aborted fetuses for transplantation, abortion may be sought for these purposes. Late abortion is an issue because it may cause adverse effects on the mother's health and because a fetus older than 28 weeks is given the status of human being. The Chinese Ministry of Health promulgated in the 1960s a regulation to prohibit the abortion of a fetus older than 28 weeks. Late abortion not only involves multiparous women, but also involves unmarried girls who are pregnant. Both groups make every effort to hide the truth at the first stage of pregnancy. Now the rate of sexual relations and pregnancy among the unmarried is higher than it was. This increase is due to changes in the sexual behavior patterns of young people. Unfortunately, changes in the ethical environment lags behind this behavioral change. In

addition, sex education and contraceptives are not so accessible to young people.[14]

Many Chinese officials and scholars now worry about the fact that the quality of life of the entire population is deteriorating. In many villages, all of the villagers are relatives with the same surname, bringing about for some of them the label "idiot village." In these communities no person can be found intelligent enough to be responsible for the management of the village, so many subsidies are granted by the government every year. The number of handicapped is estimated at about 50 million, but the criteria according to which one can be classified as handicapped are more stringent than those in the United States. Since Mr. Deng Pufang took the position of president of the Chinese Association for the Handicapped, conditions relating to the handicapped have greatly improved. But it still may be a long time before the handicapped are integrated into societal life. Social support for their care is minimal, so the burden has to be imposed upon the family. According to our study, the cost of care for a handicapped child is about 60 percent of a worker's average salary and one parent must resign from his or her job to look after the child at home. Some handicapped children are mistreated and abused. Now they can enter colleges and universities, but they still experience discrimination in the workplace. So the idea of improving the quality of life for the entire population and preventing the birth of handicapped children is in the best interests of society, of the family, and of the handicapped person herself or himself within the current social and economic conditions of China. This way of thinking brought about the draft of the Eugenic Law and the Law of Compulsory Sterilization for the Mentally Retarded in Ganshu and Liaoning Provinces.

Health Care System

The Chinese health care system is a mixture. The public health care program covers roughly 200 million people. Its beneficiaries are mainly workers but also include professionals and employees in state-owned factories and institutes. Although their medical care is free, they must pay the costs of medical care for their children. All Tibetan people, however, have the privilege of free medical care. Some villages have developed cooperative health care programs. Most peasants in rural areas, owners and employees in private enterprises, and the unemployed must pay the costs of medical care by themselves. As a result, in some poor villages, especially in the remote mountainous areas, health care is not accessible. Under the public health care program, the demand for treatment always exceeds the supply. High-ranking officials have privileges regarding medical care and enjoy special treatment. Ordinary people, if they are to be treated satisfactorily or to be admitted into the hospital in time, have to get in through the back door, so to speak, by means of various channels.[9]

Currently the government is attempting to reform health care by implementing the lease-contract-responsibility system which has proven to be very successful in agriculture. Under this program, the more patients a physician treats, the more money he or she can earn. As a result, there is a kind of trust crisis in the fiduciary relationship between physicians and patients. If the physician makes an all-out effort at treatment, the patient or his or her relatives will wonder if the physician only wants to get more money from the treatment. If the physician's treatment is rather conservative, they will wonder if the physician and hospital manager want to save the scarce resources for high ranking officials or other privileged patients. In October of 1989, some economists and ethicists who have been involved in the field of medical care met with health administrators and advisors of the Ministry of Health to argue against the implementation of the lease-contract-responsibility system in health care. This meeting was also attended by the Minister of Health, Professor Chen Mingzhang.

SECTION TWO

What are the characteristics of Chinese contemporary medical ethics? It depends on which frame of reference is used. In this section I would like to describe the characteristics of Chinese contemporary medical ethics in reference to its Western counterparts. I would also like to consider modern Chinese ethics as compared with traditional Chinese medical ethics.

Euthanasia

Euthanasia, especially active euthanasia in general and that practiced in the case of seriously defective newborns and low birth weight infants, seems to be getting increased support from professionals as well as the public in China. The percentage of respondents from different social strata who support euthanasia is very high in the surveys made in various locations by different kinds of medical professionals working in varying institutes.[22] Most lawyers maintain the view that euthanasia, especially active euthanasia, violates existing Chinese laws. Most physicians and ethicists, on the other hand, seem not to reject active euthanasia. In journals and newspapers or on the radio, those who have come forward to argue against euthanasia are in the minority. Is it possible that there is a silent majority who are against euthanasia? It seems not to be the case. Although the audience who wrote to the radio station might be the segment of the public who were interested in and sensitive to this issue, in many surveys the respondents were randomly chosen. This was especially true of the survey I made in 1985 when euthanasia was not the hot topic it is now and many of those selected were hearing the term "euthanasia" for the first time.

However, would those who favored euthanasia in the survey actually withhold or withdraw the treatment? Perhaps not. Certainly the following two factors would influence his or her decision:

Economic	If the cost of medical care were to be paid by the patient, he or she and his or her family would be more likely to ask the physician to withhold or withdraw treatment. If the patient were receiving free medical care, he or she and his or her family would be more likely to ask the physician to continue the treatment.
Cultural	There have been cases in which the patient, his or her children, and the physician all said that the treatment was meaningless and suggested withdrawing it, but nobody took action. The children feared that other relatives would blame them for violating the principle of filial piety, and the physician feared that he or she could be accused of malpractice or murder.

The attitude towards newborns and towards the elderly is different from that in the United States. It is very difficult to withdraw treatment from the elderly person who is terminally ill, whereas treatment for seriously defective newborns and very low birth weight infants is easily stopped. Due to the fact that some parents even give up on babies such as those with only a hare lip or seal fin deformity, we feel it necessary to take measures to protect them. The reasons are:

Historical	Infanticide has been a traditional practice in China. As early as 300 BC, an ancient philosopher Han Fei criticized female infanticide in the book Han Fei Zi compiled by his disciples.
Economic	It is considered an unbearable burden for a young couple to raise a seriously defective newborn or a very low birth weight infant.
Cultural	Newborns with a serious deformity have been considered monsters and were labelled "monster fetuses." These babies were not accepted by the community.
Political	Under the policy of "one couple, one child," the parents tend to withdraw treatment from the child so that the one child they may raise will be healthy.

There seems to be a paradox in China: severe measures for birth control on the one hand, and arduous efforts to solve the problem of infertility on the other. Perhaps nobody in China would deny that overpopulation is one of the biggest problems and that, to solve this problem, some measures have to be taken to control the rate of population growth. A seemingly reasonable goal set by the government is to maintain the population at a level no higher than two billion by the year 2000. In China nobody has argued against the need to control the growth rate. If this cannot be done, it will create a great burden not only upon China itself but also upon its neighbors and the other countries of the world. Many people, even though they wish to have more than one child, are nevertheless content with that one because they feel they have a commitment to the welfare of the society at large.

The issue which can be argued is whether the policy of "one couple, one child" is optimal for controlling overpopulation. The optional alternatives which have been proposed are:

"One couple, one and a half children." This proposal was suggested by Professor Li, T-L, Beijing Medical University. It means that if a couple gives birth to a girl the first time, they may have the option of a second pregnancy.

"Stop after giving birth to a boy if the parents live in a rural area." This was suggested by Dr. Gu, Z-S, Shihezi Medical College Hospital, Xinjiang Autonomous Region. It means that a couple living in the countryside may continue to bear children until they have a boy.

"One couple, two and a half children if the parents live in a rural area." This was suggested by an official in the Office of Works in Rural Areas after negotiation with some peasants who want two or three children. It means that if a couple in the countryside have girls the first two times, or one girl and one boy, they may have the option of a third pregnancy.

All of these alternatives show that the issue is not whether or not reproductive rights should be limited, but rather what is the most acceptable and efficient way to affect such a limitation. However, none of these suggestions were accepted by policymakers, perhaps because they are a bit too complicated to be practical.

Recently, there was another suggestion to the effect that it would be better to take a *laissez faire* policy on the population problem. It has been argued that, following the examples of advanced countries, the people themselves will feel it necessary to limit family size in order to promote the development of the economy and provide for compulsory education. But when will the Chinese people do that? At the time when China has a population of 4, or of 10 billion population? And even then, in view of the strong adherence to Confucian tradition in China, such a general practice is unlikely. It should not be forgotten that, when Westerners criticized the practice of limiting the right to reproduction and withdrew financial support for the population development program, they did not face the fact that we were left with the very serious problem of overpopulation in China. In many cases, because of the lack of efficient contraceptives and qualified medical personnel, abortion became a final resort. Withdrawal of assistance only worsens this situation.

There is a clear difference between the attitude towards abortion in the United States and that found in the People's Republic of China. The dominant Confucian view never treats the fetus as a human being. It values the dead body, teaching that, when dying, the body should be kept intact. In the Three Teachings (Confucianism, Taoism, and Buddhism) which shaped Chinese culture, only Chinese Buddhism put any restraints on abortion because it teaches that the fetus is a form of life. According to Buddhist doctrine, the Buddhist mission is to save all forms of life "from the bitter sea to the other shore--Western paradise." Modern doctors, however, question from a different ethical perspective, that is, whether a fetus older than 28 weeks should be treated as a human being.

In this tradition, there is no problem in using tissues and organs of the aborted fetus for transplantation. On the other hand, it is very difficult to procure dead bodies and organs for medical education and transplantation because, according to one of the Confucian classics, *Book of Filial Piety*, "skin and hair cannot be damaged because they are inherited from the parents." Although the Chinese now believe that the body will be destroyed after burial, and cremation is becoming very popular in China, they still prefer keeping a body intact to using the crematorium. Medical professors have been known to ask workers or crematoria to send them corpses to dissect for educational purposes. In the capitol of Xinjiang Autonomous Region, Ulumuqi, the director of the crematorium was sued and arrested for selling corpses. Many professors or other faculty members in the Xinjiang Medical College testified that the director had only sent them the bodies of those without relatives and that they were to be used for medical education. These educators claimed that if the director of the crematorium were found guilty and sentenced to prison, they would be willing to go to jail for him.

The infertility rate of newly-married couples and their consequent behavior might be similar in China to those in other countries. But the eagerness of infertile Chinese couples may be stronger than that of couples in other countries. Under the influence of Confucianism, a man or woman without a child would bear a heavy psychological burden. One of the requirements of filial piety is to extend the life of ancestors to future generations. According to Mencius (one of the greatest Confucianists, next only to Confucius), there are three vices which violate the principle of filial piety, and the biggest of these is to be without offspring. Traditional Chinese believe that barrenness is due to lack of virtue or to the lack of virtue of one's ancestors. The burden is especially heavy for women. Infertility is always blamed on wives who are stigmatized and abused by the family as a result of failure to conceive.

How, then, ought we to reconcile between the strong emphasis on birth control and the development of reproductive technologies? There are two interpretations of the policy "one couple, one child." One interpretation is "no child is better than one." The other is "one child is better than more than one and less than one." It seems that the latter has been widely accepted. Some officials and ethicists argue that solving the problem of infertility may decrease resistance to the family limitation policy, a policy which is only a limitation and not a deprivation of the right to reproduce. The development and use of reproductive technology will promote the infertile family's happiness by assisting them in their first exercise of the basic right to reproduce.

The Chinese are worried about overpopulation as well as quality of life. Even though they are spiritual individualists in the sense that they have always been taught to actualize self-development, self-perfection, and self-improvement, they have also been taught that they are members of the larger family--

"descendants of the Red Emperor and the Yellow Emperor." They feel that they have commitments of duty to this family. Any programs which are supposed to improve the quality of life for the nation, including compulsory sterilization of the mentally retarded and negative eugenics, are acceptable to the Chinese. This might be accomplished by reducing the number of physically and mentally handicapped persons by means of genetic counseling and screening combined with administrative measures such as prohibiting marriages between close relatives. Laws might be adopted which prohibit some types of physically and mentally handicapped persons from conceiving naturally, allowing reproduction only by AID. These methods are aimed at eliminating societal burdens. They are different from Hitler's positive eugenics, which elicits a strong negative response in China as in the West.

A strong practice of paternalism has been handed down from ancient times to the present. Chinese doctors have seldom ever talked about the patient's autonomy or self-determination, except when treating powerful persons. One traditional doctor says in his book, "When the ailing themselves cannot make any decisions, I will make them in their place. I always put myself in their place."[4] Since 1949, there has been a gradual fading away of familial paternalism, and there has developed in its place a decisionmaking mechanism in hospitals which emphasizes consultation between physician and family members involving the competent patient, sometimes including the patient's close friends or co-workers and the chief of the unit in which the patient works. Roughly speaking, the medical decision is made by the family after consulting with the attending physician. In this mechanism the patient's opinion is taken under adequate consideration, but is not considered to be an exercise of his or her right to self-determination.

In the making of a medical decision, not only the patient's interest, but also the interest of her or his whole family is placed under consideration. In the case of the terminally ill, if the patient has a higher salary and enjoys free medical care, he or she may prefer lingering in bed as long as possible, even though he or she wishes to die more peacefully and painlessly. In some cases, the patient may refuse to be informed and ask the physician to provide the information only to her or his spouse or children. It means that Chinese patients traditionally do not make a strong effort to exercise the right to self-determination. But recently some changes have taken place. For example, the cases I mentioned in the beginning of this paper (that some terminally ill persons committed suicide after their request for withdrawal of treatment has been refused by their physicians) show the awakening of the sense of autonomy. In this negative way they claimed their right to self-determination. When there is a consensus on the medical decision after deliberate consideration and sufficient consultation between the patient, his or her family, and the physician, nobody intervenes if there is no financial or emotional conflict between them.

Legal intervention in medical cases has no tradition. In the premodern period, the legal system was never involved in purely medical cases unless there was some suspicion of murder. During the Nationalist regime before 1949, physicians could be sued for malpractice, but the Chinese preferred to resolve their disputes outside the legal system. They felt that presence in court was shameful. After the 1950s, the settlement of medical disputes was transferred to health administrations. But there are no laws or regulations concerning medical disputes. In addition, health administrations are so busy that the treatment of medical disputes has been extremely unsatisfactory, protecting the right of neither patient nor physician. There have been cases in which relatives of the patient thought there was malpractice and, after becoming impatient with the slow and inefficient process of dealing with their complaint by the health administration, went to the physician's office and attacked him physically to retaliate for the perceived injustice. Now, after the Cultural Revolution, the legal system is again involved in medical cases. In Shanghai there is a draft of a law concerning medical disputes which has been experimentally used in the legal system since 1988. Information on the result of this experiment has yet to be gathered.

Both legal and ethical constraints on medical malpractice are underdeveloped in China. Since 1937, there has been no medical ethical code adopted by the Chinese Medical Association. An interesting development is that of December, 1988, when the Chinese Ministry of Health drew up and promulgated a brief ethical code for medical personnel. This code instructs medical personnel to "heal the wounds, rescue the dying, practice socialist humanitarianism," to "respect the patient's personality and his or her rights, treat all equally without discrimination," and to "respect the patient's privacy and to keep his or her confidence."[6]

SECTION THREE

Contemporary Chinese medical ethics has been developed in a country with a backward economy, a power-centralized political system, a population of 1 billion--one quarter of whom are illiterate and semi-illiterate, and a cultural tradition of thousands of years. Chinese culture was shaped by the Three Teachings: Confucianism, Taoism, and Buddhism. Moral intuition as well as moral attitudes towards medical ethical issues and resolution of ethical dilemmas (at lay, professional, and societal levels) are affected by the longstanding, entrenched traditional values and the current dominant ideology. The Three Teachings provide a unique organic worldview as a conceptual framework for the explanation and treatment of disease and a unique ethics with strong virtue-oriented and deontological focus for dealing with the relationship between physicians and patients. In the final section, I will attempt to provide an explanation of these characteristics as introduced and described in Section Two. They can best be understood in terms of Chinese culture, particularly by noting the unique influence of Chinese culture upon contemporary medical ethics.

Conceptions of Life, Death, and Suffering.

In approximately the third century BC, the great Confucianist Xun Kuang and the great legalist Han Fei were said to have argued that a human being begins with birth and ends with death. Since then, this view has become a conventional Chinese view. Traditionally, the mourning period after a person's death continued for seven weeks, but a dead fetus was never mourned. There is a contradiction, however, to this traditional belief and consequent practice: when a baby is born, it is considered to be one year old. One explanation is that the Chinese emphasize the continuity between the fetus before birth and the baby after birth, but they do not necessarily hold that the fetus is a human being or a person. When the abortion, spontaneous or induced, took place, the Chinese never said that a person or human being died. One reason for this view may be, perhaps, that the premodern Chinese have never developed a technique which allowed them to understand fetal life and development; even contemporary Chinese know very little about this process.

What then is life or death? Both Confucianists and Taoists see life as the coordination of Qi (vital force), death as the dispersion of Qi. The life of a person is the product of interaction between $Yang$ (light Qi) and Yin (heavy Qi). $Yang$ comes from Heaven and father, and Yin from Earth and mother. After the death of a person, $Yang$ is returned to Heaven and Yin to Earth. So a person comes from nature and returns to it. The least intelligent being, an amoeba, and the most intelligent being, a human being, each consists of Qi, and they are integral parts of a continuum--a chain of beings which is never broken because nothing is outside of it.

Birth and death are two of the greatest events in human life, because each person only has one chance to be born and one chance to die. So the Chinese have a grand ceremony to celebrate these occasions. Birth and death are called "red and white happy events." Birth is nothing but a new form of Qi, and so is death. For Confucianism, what is valued is not human life itself, but living in an ideal way. The great historian Sima Qian said that every person must die, and that a person's death is as heavy as the Tai Mountains and as light as a feather of the wild goose. Confucius once said: "A man of humanity will never seek to live at the expense of injuring humanity. He would rather sacrifice his life in order to realize humanity."[2] What is valued is a meaningful, not a meaningless life. The meaning of life for Confucianists is found by following Confucian ethical principles which teach people to be human--to be worthy members of the universal family. Moreover, for Confucianists, to live or to die is not a thing which can be controlled by human beings. Confucius once said: "Life and death are the chance of Heaven; wealth and honor depend on Heaven."[2]

For Taoists, one school emphasizes the preserving of life by means of breathing properly, exercise, diet, sex, and appropriate medicines. What Taoists want to preserve is a natural existence in which will be maintained a harmony or balance of Yin and $Yang$ within the human body and between it and the universe.

For the major Taoists, an ideal spiritual sphere for a human being is to transcend all distinctions or dichotomies including life and death. Why should we be pleasant at birth and sad at death? And the great Taoist Zhuang Zhou once said that the most unhappy thing in the world is mind-death, because then a person becomes a walking corpse.

For Chinese Buddhists, the highest goal a person can reach is Nirvana in which life and death are transcended. In this state all things in their own nature are truly experienced as unreal and void. To reach Nirvana and save all forms of life, it is necessary for a person to get rid of *karmas* and return to the emptiness of original mind.

As for suffering, Confucianists see it as the tempering of one's moral character. As Mencius said: "When Heaven is about to confer a great responsibility on any man, it will exercise his mind with sufferings, subject his sinews and bones to hard work, expose his body to hunger, put him to poverty, place obstacles in the paths of his deeds, so as to stimulate his mind, harden his nature, and improve wherever he is incompetent."[2]

The Three Teachings have developed a doctrine to help the Chinese release themselves from suffering. There are two elements in this doctrine. The one is "non-action" (*Wu Wei*) which does not mean "do nothing," but rather do nothing unnaturally or beyond nature. One source of suffering is that which one desires to be rather than that which nature permits. The other is attachment. One can pursue something, seek for something, but must not be attached to it. If one is non- or de-attached and something that has been gained is lost one day, it will not cause any suffering to her or him. When a patient is terminally ill, why do we prolong his or her dying unnaturally? Why do we attach to this existence which is going to cease naturally? Let nature take its course. For Chinese Buddhists especially, suffering is caused by failing to know the truth that all things in the universe are nothing more than the apparent phenomena of mental activities; by keeping the mind in a state of emptiness and calmness, all suffering can be avoided.

The Chinese conceptions of life, death, and suffering have led them to the following attitude: Treasure human life but do not attach to it. The suffering experienced by the Chinese has been, perhaps, much greater than that experienced by any other nation but, by this attitude, the Chinese have been able to cope with the burden of death and release themselves from it.

Holistic Socio-Political Philosophy

A quasi-holistic socio-political philosophy has been developed from Chinese cultural tradition. It is based on two thousand years of power-centralized, autocratic monarchy--one that has lacked any rights-oriented, individualistic, liberal democratic tradition. In recent decades, Marxism--rather, a mixture of Russian and Chinese versions of Marxism--has become the dominant ideology. The historicism and social holism of this system, interwoven with traditional ideas, puts the greatest emphasis on nation, society, and country rather than on individuals.

In ancient China there were two factors which exerted far-reaching influence upon Chinese socio-political philosophy. One was ancestor worship, the other was the patriarchal clan system. Both of these imply respect for the elderly. In the patriarchal clan system, all members of a community are looked upon as blood related or kin-related in one way or another. The consequence is that family is seen as the model of society or country. This is a duty-oriented model, in which each member has his or her own role responsibilities: children have the duty of filial piety to their parents, parents have the duty of kindness to their children. There are also similar reciprocal duties between husband and wife, brothers and sisters, friends, ruler and subjects, superior and inferior, teacher and student, physician and patient, and so on.

Although the relationship between the members of each pair is reciprocal, they are not equal. The father, husband, and ruler always play a guiding role in their relationships with son, wife, and subject. The authority figure in a family or clan is the patriarch; in a country it is the ruler--the patriarch of the country. In this system, all the decisions about family or state affairs are made by the patriarch, the head of the family, or the head of the country. In premodern China, a county magistrate was called "parental official of the county." Now, however, patriarchal authority is in decline. Decisions involving the family still need to be made by all members of the family after consultation, not by any one individual.

I have mentioned that the Chinese are spiritually individualistic in the sense that they always pay a considerable amount of attention to self-development and self-perfection. Mencius illustrated this in the solution he provided to a hypothesized dilemma presented by him to his disciples in a thought experiment. The dilemma is: "If the safe-king Shun's father, the Old Blind Man, had committed murder, and the honest man Gae Yao had been appointed as the Minister of Justice, what ought Shun to do?"

Mencius's solution is: "Shun ought to resign from the position of the Son of Heaven (king), take his father out of jail stealthily, escape with him to a mountain, and support him up to his end."

Mencius's solution to this dilemma shows that he gave the priority to the principle of filial piety which ought to be developed before all others. But in later periods, Confucianists advocated the meta-principle of "loyalty first, filial piety second." And since the Song Dynasty when neo-Confucianists upheld the preservation of heavenly principles and the elimination of human desires, the Chinese have gradually lost their atomistic character, and have become instead water droplets in an ocean.

Marx defined the essence of a human being as the sum of social relations. For Marxists, society is more than the sum of individuals and, consequently, societal institutions and their changes cannot be explained in terms of individual human actions. Chinese Marxists always describe the relationship between individuals, collectives, and country as that between leaves, branches, and root. Marxist social holism implies that individual interests should be subordinated to public interests. And Marxist historicism implies that it is necessary for human beings to sacrifice the not-so-happy present for the future happy life. When Chinese traditional quasi-holistic, socio-political philosophy is combined with Marxist holism, there is an exponential effect which leads to the strong statement: Rights-oriented individualism is essentially alien to the Chinese.

However, with the advance of modernization, the phenomenon I call "the awakening of the rights sense" can be observed: students and intellectuals are striving for civil rights, girls in villages are claiming the right to freely chosen marriages (as opposed to accepting arranged marriages), and patients are asserting the right to self-determination.

Chinese Ethics: A Unique Virtue-Oriented and Deontological Ethics with Weak Normative Aspects

Chinese ethics may be said to be the expression of the discovery of what it is to be a human being. We are born human in the biological sense, but we are badly in need of discovering what it means to be human in the moral sense. For a Chinese, the statement: You are not human! is a very serious epithet. The uniqueness of being human cannot be reduced to biological, psychological, or sociological structures and functions because a living person is far more complex and meaningful than a momentary instance of existence. Inherent in the structure of the human is the infinite potential for development. However, the actual process of this development or self-cultivation cannot be separated from ordinary human experience and daily life. For Confucianists, humaneness (ren) or loving others is what distinguishes humans from animals. This is the primary moral duty. For Confucianists, humaneness should be practiced from the near to the far, beginning with filial piety. They emphasize that the practice of humaneness arises in the agent's inner heart, and it is useless to impose ethical or legal constraints from outside without the cultivation of this virtue in the heart. As Confucius said: "The achieving of humanenss depends upon oneself; how can (it depend) upon others? If a man is not humane, what is the use of knowing norms?"[18]

The basis of being human, as Mencius argues, is in the inner structure of human nature--human nature as good. A human being is born with four seeds: the heart of commiseration, the heart of shame and dislike, the heart of deference and compliance, and the heart of right and wrong. These are developed by self-cultivation into the four virtues of humaneness, righteousness, propriety, and wisdom, respectively. Why does a human being do evil? Because his or her original mind was obstructed by selfish desires and external forces. So self-cultivation consists of searching for the lost original mind. Much of the later work done by Chinese philosophers concentrated on how to find the original mind, that is, on self-cultivation.

This approach has had a far-reaching influence upon Chinese medical ethics. As I have explained in an article on traditional medicine,[10] Chinese medical ethicists have always emphasized that medicine is the art of humaneness. The focus of this art is the search for ways to cultivate the heart of humaneness in medical personnel by rectifying themselves. This emphasis has resulted in neglect of the social control of medical knowledge by ethical and legal constraints.

However, medical ethics has become one of the most flourishing disciplines in China at a time when China is changing from a monolithic country into a rather pluralistic one. We are now encountering the historical period of so-called modernization (a paradigm shift period indeed!) during which the Chinese want to condense the Renaissance, the Reformation, the Enlightenment and the Industrial Revolution in a matter of decades. There are, and will continue to be, conflicts and tensions between different, incompatible, or even incommensurable values in all fields. This tends to make everything uncertain and changeable, both in public life and the field of medical care. The only reasonable way of resolving these conflicts and tensions between different social and cultural groups is through continuing dialogue, consultation, and negotiation between different social and cultural groups.

NOTES

1   Cai G.F., et al. A preliminary approach to the problems of medical ethics. *Medicine and Philosophy*, 1980;2:44-48.
2   Chan W.T. *A Source Book on Chinese Philosophy*. Princeton, NJ:Princeton University Press, 1963;43.
3   Guo Q.X., et. al. A survey on euthanasia. *Medicine and Philosophy*, 1988;6:34-36.
4   Huai Yuan. *A Thorough Understanding of Medicine in Ancient and Modern Times*, 1936. The name and location of the publishing house are not mentioned in the book.
5   Ma, An, *et al*. A preliminary analysis of the present situation of China's population. *Population Research*, 1984;3:8.
6   People's Daily, 1988 December 12;1. See also *Chinese Hospital Management* 1989;9(no.3):5.
7   Qiu R.Z. A report on the First National Conference on Social, Ethical, and Legal Issues in Euthanasia. *Studies in Dialectics of Nature*, 1988;6:61-63.
8   Qiu R.Z. AID confronts the law in China. *Hastings Center Report*, 1989;6: 3-4.
9   Qiu R.Z. Equity and public health care in China. *The Journal of Philosophy*, 1989;283-288.
10   Qiu R.Z. Medicine--the art of humaneness: On the ethics of traditional Chinese medicine. *The Journal of Medicine and Philosophy*, 1988;13:277-300.

11   Qiu R.Z. Philosophy of medicine in the 1970's. In: *Studies in Philosophy of Science*, Beijing:The Knowledge Press, 1982;281-331.

12   Qiu R.Z. The concepts of death and euthanasia. *Medicine and Philosophy*, 1980;1:77-79.

13   Qiu R.Z, *et al*. A survey on bioethics. *Medicine and Philosophy*, 1988;6: 34-36.

14   Qiu R.Z, *et. al*. Can late abortion be ethically justified? *The Journal of Philosophy*, 1989;14:343-350.

15   Sass H.M., ed. *Case Studies for Bioethical Diagnosis*. Zentrum fur Medizinnishe Ethik:Ruhr-Universitat Bochum, 1989;1.

16   Sun Simiao. *The Important Prescriptions Worth a Thousand Pieces of Gold*. Printed in the period of Wanli's reign, Ming Dynasty. Volume 1;9-11.

17   Unschuld P. *Medical Ethics in Imperial China--A Study in Historical Anthropology*, Berkeley,CA:UC Press, 1979;102.

18   Wang J. The new document of medical ethics. *Chinese Journal of Medicine*, 1944;30:39-40.

19   Ware J.R., trans. *The Sayings of Confucius*. New York: Mentor Books, 1955;76,129. There is some change in the quoted English translation.

20   According to the estimate by participants of the First National Conference on Social, Ethical, and Legal Issues in Reproductive Technology held in Yueyang, Hunan Province in November 1989. The proceedings are not available.

21   Read at the First International Conference on the Future of Medicine: The Western and Eastern Perspectives 2000. Bad Homburg: Federal Republic of Germany 1989(March). The proceedings have not yet been published.

22   At the First National Conference on Social, Ethical, and Legal Issues in Euthanasia, many papers were submitted which reported the results of these surveys.

13

Ancient and Modern Medical Ethics in India

C. M. Francis

INTRODUCTION

India ranks as the second most populous country and the largest democracy in the world. In 1988, it had an estimated population of 818.8 million. Its rich cultural heritage is a rational synthesis of ancient Indian thought, philosophy, and ethics. This concrescence, which has continued to develop as is gathers new concepts, has kept pace with current thought and has never been remote from popular understanding.

The basis of India's cultural history is found primarily in spiritual experience and secondarily in *dharma* (ethical conduct according to one's state), as these are the two most important concepts of Indian thought. In addition, the dynamic cultural heritage often influences and sometimes confronts new thinking, especially that originating in other cultures.

Dr. S. Radhakrishnan, a former President of India and Professor of Oriental philosophy at the University of Oxford says:

> Reverence for the past is a national trait. There is a certain doggedness of temperament, a stubborn loyalty to lose nothing in the long march of the ages. When confronted with new culture or sudden extensions of knowledge, the Indian does not yield to the temptations of the hour, but holds fast to his traditional faith, importing as much as possible of the new into the old. Conservative liberalism is the secret of the success of India's culture and civilization.[15]

Though India's value systems have been influenced by all of the country's religions, Hinduism dominates as the major religion. It is practiced by 82.64 percent of the people, contributing to the development of practical philosophy and ethics. These ethics are based on the Hindu belief that we are all part of the divine Paramatman: we have in each of us Atman, part of that Paramatman. The ultimate aim is for our Atman to coalesce with Paramatman or Brahman to become one.

According to the Vedas (4000 BC to 1000 BC), the call to love one's neighbor as oneself is a response to the understanding that "thy neighbor is in truth thy very self and what separates you from him is mere illusion (*maya*)." Hence the conduct of a doctor (like that of any other person) will be motivated by agapic love and will. As a result, the relationship will be ethically sound: the patient and the doctor are part of the same unity.

Closely allied with Hinduism are Jainism and Buddhism. These religions proclaim: *ahimsa paramo dharma*. Most important of all, our actions must be *ahimsa*, usually translated as non-violence, which was enunciated by Buddha and practiced by Gandhiji to obtain political freedom. However, the Indian traditional concept of *ahimsa* goes beyond non-violence. Patanjali defined this as "*Sarvatha Sarvada sarvabutanam anabhidroha*--a complete absence of ill-will to all beings."

Ayurveda, the ancient science of life, lays down the principles for management of health and disease and for the physician's code of conduct. Charaka[10] described the objectives of medicine as two-fold: (1) the preservation of good health and, (2) combating disease (*swasthaduraparayanam cha*). How close to the emerging vision of the role of the physician! Ayurveda emphasizes the need for a healthy lifestyle which includes cleanliness and purity, good diet, proper behavior, and mental and physical discipline. This is carried out by proper *dinacharya* (daily routine) and *rtucharya* (according to seasons). One must observe purity and cleanliness in everything: *jalasuddi* (pure water), *aharasuddi* (clean food), *dehasuddi* (clean body), *manasuddi* (pure mind), and *desasuddi* (environment). Ayurveda is a science of health which is more inclusive than the science of curing diseases and the otherwise ill.

Ayurveda calls upon the physician to treat the patient as a whole:

Dividho jayate vyadih
Sariro manasasthatha
Parasparam tayorjanma
Nirdvandvam nopalabhyate

                    Aswamedha parva of Mahabharata

[Diseases occur both physically and mentally and even though one part might be dominant, it cannot be compartmentalized and separated from the whole].

The ancient Ayurvedic system, influenced by the Upanishads, treats man as a unity--body, mind, and what is beyond mind. The earliest proponents of Indian medicine, including Atreya, Kashyapa, Bhela, Charaka, and Susruta, have based their writings on foundations of spiritual philosophy and ethics formulated by the ancient *rshis* (sages). But the single teacher of Ayurveda who established this science on the foundation of spirituality and ethics was Vagbhata, the author of *Astanga Hridaya*.[16] Vagbhata says:

Sukarthah sarvabutanam
Matah sarvah pravrthayah
Sukham ca na vina dharmat
thasmad dharmaparo bhavet.

[All activities of man are directed to the end of attaining happiness, whereas happiness is never achieved without righteousness. It is the strict duty of man to be righteous in his action.]

Vagbhata further declares that it is the duty of every man to serve, to the best of his ability, those who are afflicted, even the lowliest creatures.

Charaka Samhita developed an elaborate code of conduct which can be simply stated: The medical profession must be motivated by compassion for all living beings (*bhuta-daya*).[17] His humanistic ideal became evident in his advice to physicians.[10]

He who practices not for money nor for caprice but out of compassion for living beings (*bhuta-daya*), is the best among all physicians. It is difficult to find a conferor of religious blessings comparable to the physician who snaps the snares of death for his patients. The physician who regards compassion for living beings as the highest religion fulfills his mission (*siddharthah*) and obtains the highest happiness.

Medical ethics in India today is in flux because of the impact of developments in the West on ancient concepts and because of changes in the socioeconomic situation. Problems have arisen mainly in the following categories:

- Those concerning professional activities of doctors and related professionals--such as the ethics of trust versus the ethics of rights, and informed consent and rights of patients versus paternalism.
- Those connected with social justice and equity--issues such as equal access to treatment by sophisticated technology, controls of experiments on human beings, and the right of all to basic health care.
- Those related mainly to the beginning and end of life--issues such as the propriety of IVF and termination of life support, and the right to life.

INFORMED CONSENT

Doctors in India generally believe that informed consent cannot be obtained because of rampant illiteracy. They think that patients are unable to make a reasoned choice because of their inability to appreciate the intricacies of alternative medical treatment, procedures, or drug trials. Often a paternalistic view is taken: The doctor knows best. Providing information has proven troublesome and time-consuming. Doctors reason: Why take the trouble to attempt to inform when the patient will agree anyway to whatever the doctor suggests? Is consent not implicit in the very fact that the patient has sought the expertise of the doctor?

Dr. Srinivasamurthy and his colleagues[20] at the National Institute of Mental Health and Neurosciences, Bangalore, conducted a study of the relevance of obtaining informed consent. Nearly all (99 percent) of the participants in a drug trial made clearly expressed decisions as to whether or not they wanted to participate. Their choices were based on the adequacy of the information supplied which, in turn, was relative to their capacity to understand and deliberate. These capacities did not correlate with social, economic, educational, or other background characteristics.

Ought the doctor to withhold treatment if it is not possible to obtain informed consent? There seems to be a conflict between the moral duty of the doctor to act beneficently and the legal right of a patient to understand and agree to every treatment. According to present law in India, a person is not allowed to commit suicide. But is it morally justifiable for an individual to refuse medical treatment and thus forfeit saving his own life? Will the doctor be assisting suicide if he or she does not do all that is possible to prevent a suicide attempt from being successful? On the other hand, does not the patient have the right to determine what shall be done to his or her body?

Another question of concern is: What would be the place of informed consent if a patient were admitted to the hospital in critical condition but with senses still fully intact? Could the surgeon who diagnosed the condition as one requiring immediate surgery, refuse to operate on the sole ground that the patient had not given consent for the operation? If the patient died due to the physician's refusal to perform the surgery, what would be the doctor's liability be?

Recently, an interesting case occurred in the State of Kerala. A man with acute abdominal pain was admitted to a government hospital. The duty doctor examined him and diagnosed his condition as perforated appendix with general peritonitis, a condition which required an immediate operation. But the surgeon did not operate and the patient died the next day. The patient's dependents filed suit against the doctor and the Kerala government for damages. The defense argued that the patient's consent was necessary before the doctor could operate and, since the patient did not give it, the operation was not done. The court rejected this plea and granted a decree against the doctor personally, absolving the government, however. The Kerala High Court upheld the judgment in an appeal filed by the doctor.

Two surgeons who were called as expert witnesses stated that they would have operated on the patient without explicit consent. Dr. A. Ramaswamy Iyengar, Director, R .V. Institute of Sanskrit Studies (personal communications) testified: "Informed consent of patients is not required. Faith in the doctor is more important on the part of a patient than his intellectual compliance or otherwise." This is the general view of the public and the majority of doctors in India today.

In contrast to the above, there is another view which holds that every human being has a right to determine what shall be done with his or her own body; a surgeon who performs an operation without the patient's consent thereby commits an assault for which he is liable.[13] Angela Roddey Holder maintains that, "In the medical context, the mere fact that one puts oneself into the hands of physicians does not mean that they can proceed as they see fit. They have a duty to explain what sort of treatment they propose and why and to point out significant risks or reasonable alternatives. They also have a legal duty to limit treatment to that to which one has consented. If they go beyond the boundaries, even for the patient's good and with good results, physicians violate the patient's right."[8]

Indian physicians who are trained abroad or who have accepted this principle find themselves in a situation of conflict. What is the ancient teaching in such circumstances? Charaka advises the physician to take into confidence the close relatives, the elders in the community, and even the state officials before undertaking procedures which might end in the patient's death. The physician should then proceed with the treatment.

In India, the "ethics of trust" (trust of the physician's judgment) has been and continues to be in vogue. But more and more people are questioning the practice. They want to make their own decisions, especially in the light of what is happening in the West. They are not willing to accept mistakes, even those made inadvertently. The old idea of accepting philosophically any harm done and attributing it to *karma*, or fate, is fading. The "ethics of trust" based on the "goodness" of the doctor is slowly giving way to the "ethics of rights" based on an assertion of the individual's right to decide for himself or herself.

UNETHICAL TREATMENT

It is a common experience to become aware of dramatic examples of unethical practices; often they are found in media advertising. In both developing and developed countries, instances of unethical practices can be seen in unsubstantiated claims for treatment. Many people, hopeful of being cured and looking for any chance of relief, try these treatments which lack scientific validity. One example is a recent case at King's College Hospital in London in which a hematologist and a veterinarian claimed without basis to have developed immunotherapy against AIDS.

In the matter of unethical treatment, it has been stated that the difference between the developed countries and the developing countries is similar to the difference between capitalism and socialism. But this claimed divergence is probably best expressed by the following comment: There is a big difference. Under capitalism, man exploits man. Under socialism, it is the other way round. It seems, however, that unsubstantiated claims for cures are most common in India, with its mass of illiterate and gullible people. Some doctors take advantage of this situation by promoting these "cures." Other doctors, who are aware of such charlatan practices, share responsibility because they do not expose them. It is clear that the ancients frowned upon such practices.

UNETHICAL ADVERTISEMENTS

Few instances occur concerning unethical advertisements by doctors. Colleagues frown upon such advertisements, though little action follows. The Medical Council is responsible for looking into such matters, but the doctor often escapes on technicalities.

Recently, advertisements by hospitals and diagnostic centers have become highly visible, claiming that their institution is superior to others. This is creating problems. "It is totally unethical. I think any agency worth its name will not advertise in such a manner," says Joe D'Silva, General Manager of Imageads.[3] Mr. Vikram Reddy, Creative Director at R.K. Swamy, says, "If I were heading an agency, I would not resort to such unhealthy advertising." Since it is the general trend in the country in all commercial industrial advertising, however, competitive advertising is bound to be adopted by the "health industry." There is little guidance from the ancients on this topic because there were no advertisements in their time.

DIAGNOSTIC AIDS

There is a growing supermarket in diagnostic equipment. Sophisticated equipment is bought by third world countries at great expense, using scarce foreign currency. Most of the imaging equipment currently in use in various hospitals and diagnostic laboratories is excessive when related to the needs of the population and the complexity of operation and maintenance. When funds are put into high technology, the great majority of people cannot have the benefit of even the most elementary x-ray examinations.

Third world countries are sometimes used as dumping grounds for equipment not needed elsewhere or for substandard diagnostic aids withdrawn from developed countries. A poignant example was the sale of defective diagnostic kits for AIDS. India is experiencing serious problems because it was not cautious enough in ordering AIDS kits from a West German multinational corporation. These kits were substandard and produced many false negatives. India's entire AIDS control program has been in jeopardy because the kits were unreliable. And it masked the extent of the prevalence of AIDS in the country. Inquiries to the West German control authority revealed that the lot of kits supplied to India (including those supplied to the Indian Council of Medical Research) were those recalled from the European market early in 1988.

Yet another problem with the purchase of equipment from abroad has been the difficulty with servicing and maintenance. Indian doctors trained abroad in sophisticated procedures often order costly equipment they have used in the countries of their training. The aspirations of these specialists are understandable, but should these not be tempered by the realities of the situation? The equipment may function for some time, but when it goes out of order, there is no backup service. The net result is that the equipment lies idle and the doctor is unable to do diagnoses according to the methods in which he or she was trained.

The questions are: Is it ethical for the doctor to order costly, sophisticated equipment, which is not likely to function, utilizing scarce foreign currency? Is it ethical for firms to supply these items without back-up service? This is a problem in most third world countries. Thairu[21] suggests that "an ethical code should be agreed on by both (manufacturers and users) regarding the sale of equipment."

DRUGS AND PHARMACEUTICALS

There is a huge proliferation of drugs in the Indian market, with more than 60,000 formulations. Multinational and national factories, ranging from tin-shed to large operations, manufacture the drugs. Many of the small factories work on the basis of "loan licenses" from the large firms. These small scale industries are not subject to stringent rules and regulations. The larger firms then market the product under their brand name.

Many drugs in the Indian market have been banned in other countries. Some drugs which were banned in India itself continue to be marketed after obtaining stay orders from the courts. Because legal proceedings take such a long time, doctors can continue to prescribe these hazardous drugs to patients, and firms continue to make huge profits.

As previously mentioned, many drugs on the market are useless or of substandard quality. Although reports show, as a rule, twenty to thirty percent of the samples tested are substandard, multinational and national firms continue to manufacture these products. Government agencies take a long time to test the samples and to release their findings. Long before the announcement, a particular batch of drugs will have been prescribed by doctors and taken by patients; many will not be aware of the announcement because often the notice is placed in a local newspaper, whereas the drug is sold countrywide. Most manufacturers do not recall the banned products. They are expected to give the indications, contraindications, side effects and adverse effects of all drugs. They often do so, but in such a way that it will not attract attention. The rule of thumb seems to be: The greater the hazard, the smaller the print.

In the *ICSSR-ICMR Study on Health for All: An Alternative Strategy*, this issue is addressed:

One of the most distressing aspects of the present health situation in India is the doctor's habit of overprescribing or prescribing glamorous and costly drugs with limited medical potential. It is also unfortunate that the drug producers try to push doctors into using their products by all means--fair or foul. These basic facts are more responsible for distortions in drug production and consumption than anything else. If the medical profession could be made to be more discriminating in its prescribing habits, there would be no market for irrational and unnecessary drugs.[9]

Drug firms generally do not follow the WHO ethical criteria for drug promotion. Giftgiving remains rampant and raises as many ethical issues as it does in other countries;[2] the harmful effects, however, are more pronounced and longer lasting in poor countries.

In the ancient days, medicines were prepared in India (as elsewhere in the world) under the personal supervision of the physician or by the families of patients. There were strict guidelines for the collection of the herbs and other raw materials and for the preparative processes. Medicines thus prepared were reliable as regards quality and purity. Today, even Ayurvedic medicines are processed on a commercial scale and what applies to modern pharmaceuticals applied equally to Ayurvedic drugs.

RIGHT TO HEALTH

Article 25 of the *Universal Declaration of Human Rights* states: "Everyone has the right to a standard of living adequate for the health and well-being of himself and of his family, including food, clothing, housing and medical care and necessary social services." If health is considered a fundamental human right, it becomes the basic responsibility of the state to protect and promote the health of all the people. A minimum of level health care services should be available to all. The state has a duty to provide this and to assure it legally.

The Alma-Ata Conference called for a new approach to health care which would close the gap between the "haves" and "have nots." Governments must achieve a more equitable distribution of health care resources and attain a level of health for all citizens of the world that will permit them to lead socially and economically productive lives. The main declaration of the conference proclaimed: "Governments have a responsibility for the health of the people, which can be fulfilled only by adequate and equitably distributed health and social measures."

The right to health brings up another issue, that of fair distribution of health care delivery: to make care available, acceptable, and affordable to all. One important aspect of fair distribution is the need for qualified health care personnel to provide services where they are unavailable. But can the physician be compelled to provide service to areas otherwise unable to obtain medical services? Can rural service be required? The state and educational institutions generally subsidize medical education. Even if there is no subsidy, the doctor has been provided an opportunity for education which is not available to many. St. John's Medical College, Bangalore, has made it mandatory that its medical graduates serve for a minimum period of two years in an underserved rural area. A few other medical colleges in the country also require that their medical graduates practice for a period of time in underserved areas. But objections arise. Since a doctor is not owned by the people or the institution, can he or she be deprived of the right to earn legitimately as much as possible, in a region of his or her choice? Can a person be compelled to act against his or her wish as long as no harm is done to society? The consensus is that, even though the medical profession, in general, does not favor mandatory service, a physician has the duty to serve people in the areas where the need is greatest.

Although health is not a fundamental human right under the Indian Constitution, the subject is included in the Directive Principles of State Policy, which is considered the "conscience" of the Indian Constitution. Article 39 of the constitution directs that state policy must ensure health care; Article 47 requires that the improvement of public health be among the primary duties of the state. In pursuance of these articles, the government has issued a number of policy statements and programs. Parliament approved the latest in the series, the National Health Policy (1982), at the end of 1983.

What rights do patients have? An estimated 25 million children in India go blind each year for want of care. This is mainly due to vitamin A deficiency. Many of these children die within weeks of becoming blind. Even children with milder forms of Vitamin A deficiency succumb to infections and malnutrition. Do they have the right to be protected against this deficiency? About 300 million people live in areas with iodine-deficient soil. The government is belatedly taking action to provide iodized salts. Doctors in the country had known for a long time about the iodine deficiency diseases--endemic goitre, cretinism, and others, but they did not raise their voices in a call for action to prevent the deficiency. And this is only one example. Millions suffer from other deficiencies and communicable diseases, often caused by failings of the society in which they live, and by lack of active concern on the part of the government and the people, including members of the medical profession.

HEALTH POLICY

There can be little objection to the stated health policy of India's government. But when it comes to implementing the policy, that is another story. The allocation of resources to the health sector has been very small. Often, the assignment of priorities is not based on the needs of the people but on what is fashionable.

An outstanding example of this neglect is understood by a comparison of the efforts made to find cures for what may be described as the diseases of affluence and for the diseases of poverty. The country's needs remain primarily those of prevention and management of diseases of malnutrition and infection. But most public money is spent to obtain sophisticated gadgets and to develop centers for treatment of degenerative cardiovascular and renal diseases. There are at least forty centers for open heart surgery. Little is made available to manage the infectious diseases which take a major toll with respect to morbidity and mortality. A prime example in recent times is kala-azar in the villages of Bihar, Orissa, and West Bengal. The whole east coast of India is vulnerable to resurgent attacks of kala-azar, a disease caused by Leishmania donovani. The efforts to prevent this disease and manage the outbreak have been poor. This has also been the case with other common communicable diseases.

Questions arise: Who shall receive which type of health care? What resources can be allocated? How? To whom? How do we set our priorities? What is an acceptable form of health care? Who should decide on health policy?

These and many other issues are being debated currently. There is a movement toward a more equitable distribution of the benefits of medical knowledge. But against it is the much more powerful force for the use of sophisticated, spectacular, and costly technology for the benefit of the few.

Newer gadgets, machinery, and technology are multiplying the expenses for diagnostic and therapeutic procedures. People are directly and indirectly pressured through various media to go through a whole array of expensive diagnostic procedures. Patients are made to feel that, unless they go through all the sophisticated tests, a correct diagnosis is not possible. P.E.S. Palmer writes: "Moving from reasonable diagnostic accuracy to near 100 percent certainty is so expensive that the business creed of cost-effectiveness is of major importance and is already clashing with the physician's ethical wish to do the best for each individual, regardless of income. That last 10 percent of accuracy often accounts for 90 percent of the cost and does not necessarily bring an equivalent benefit to the patient."[14] There are wide networks of costly diagnostic laboratories of this sort, aided and abetted by doctors, who often get kickbacks.

Patients are completely mystified by the advice they get from their physicians and the advertisements by the laboratories. They pay huge sums of money (relative to their earnings) which they can ill afford. The ethical onus rests squarely on the medical profession. In the words of Professor Ramalingaswamy,[18] the dictum should be "maximum benefit to the patient with minimum hazards and cost."

Does an individual have the right to authorize purchase of expensive technology when it will exclude others from adequate health care who share the same resources? Should a person, as an individual, because he has the money or is sponsored by the state as a result of political or economic power or influence, be able to seek and receive sophisticated technology not available to others in less fortunate circumstances? Is it right that the scarce resources of qualified and experienced personnel, as well as money--including foreign currency and goods --be used for the benefit of a few while the majority of people are not able to get even simple health care services?

All religions advocate care of the poor and needy. Christ declared: "When you have done this to the least of my brothers, you have done it to me." Gandhiji said: "I will give you a talisman. Whenever you are in doubt or when the self becomes too much with you, apply the following test: recall the face of the poorest and weakest man you have seen and ask yourself if the step you are contemplating is going to be of any use to him. Will he gain anything by it?" This was not the ancient way of thinking. Physicians were enjoined to give special care to the health needs of kings and those in authority. But Kabir on Justice in Guru Granth Sahib said: "The valiant fighter is only he who fights for justice to the poor."

Changes in the concept of providing health care are taking place throughout the world. The Alma-Ata Declaration of Health for All is one such example of the beginning of change and India is a signatory to the declaration. Oregon, in the United States, has recently considered the need to advance the health of the population as a whole versus doing everything for each individual patient. Legislators have decided to cut off Medicaid funds for organ transplants and to use the money thus saved to extend basic services.[6]

The debate goes on: Shall the state purchase twelve renal dialysis machines which will maintain the life of a few sick people, or employ fifty community health workers to help 50,000 people achieve better health? Shall the hospital buy one lithotripter or expand its program for oral rehydration for children affected with diarrhea? The cake is small; how shall it be cut?

Has the medical profession any ethical responsibility for influencing health policy? Doctors in India are often passive spectators in the fight for social justice and against discrimination in health care.

CONTROL OF FERTILITY

The government of India and the people of the country are concerned with the increase in population. The government, believing the benefits of economic development are lost because of excessive population growth, wants to control this growth by any means.

One method proposed is that of incentives and disincentives, incentives to those who subject themselves to sterilization and disincentives to those who are not willing to undergo sterilization. One example is indicated as follows: "Green card lure: the Bihar Health Department has announced that it will issue green cards to couples with two or less children and who have undergone sterilization after April 1975. The cards are to be a ticket to top priority in education, health, and housing."

Such discrimination raises an ethical issue. Why should a third or fourth child suffer from handicaps in obtaining education and other resources rather than their older siblings? The educational and other facilities in the country, especially in the villages, are limited. Favoring one works out to be discrimination against the other.

The majority of leaders in the country consider that population control is necessary. The difference in opinion is with respect to methods. Dalawari, a Sikh leader in personal communication, states: "If family planning is required, as it certainly is, artificial methods of contraception are inevitable." Swami Rangananthananda, head of the Ramkrishna ashram, Hyderabad (personal communications) adds, "It is essential to control population growth effectively. All methods for control of population growth can be used."

But a minority of others do not subscribe to this theory regarding population explosion. According to Dr. Ravi Duggal,[5] the "population bomb" is a myth. Demographers and economists present a simple conclusion that the high rate of population growth is responsible for an adverse standard of living. The government accepts this theory completely because it has to explain unemployment, poverty, disease, pestilence, and general misery. Dr. Ravi Duggal does not agree. According to Dr. Duggal, the population of India, like that of other developing countries, will stabilize as soon as the spurt in growth disappears and industrial development has declined, just as we have seen happen in the affluent countries.

Even when artificial contraception is not practiced, certain medical procedures resulting in contraception may be performed in some situations. In these cases, the primary motive would be to provide full protection for the patient.

This can be understood in the context of considering certain problems which are peculiar to under-development and lack of adequate medical care. There may be women in whom the uterus is beginning to rupture (or has already ruptured) by the time that they seek and get medical help. This condition is due to inadequate health care services. The child is delivered and then the option presents itself to do a hysterectomy or tubectomy. The reasoning for this is that it would prevent further conception leading to possible rupture of the uterus resulting in the death of the mother, or, at least, grave consequences.

Here is the dilemma: Should the doctor do a tubectomy (a simple procedure) with the intent of preventing further conception, or should he or she perform a hysterectomy (a much more serious surgery) which also has the ultimate consequence of preventing conception?

Can sterilization be justified by valid medical indications when there is no immediate life-threatening situation? Bernard Haring[7] says: "If a competent physician can determine a full agreement with his patient that in this particular situation, a new pregnancy must be excluded now and forever because it would be thoroughly irresponsible, and, if from a medical point of view, sterilization is the best possible solution, it cannot be against the principles of medical ethics nor is it against natural law." At present, physicians in India make such a decision by taking into account the effects--present and future--on the total health of the person.

In the ancient writings, artificial methods of contraception, interfering with natural processes, were advised against. But the Upanishads (*Taithiriya*) and Dharmasutras (*Manu*) enjoin that such codes of conduct are to be determined from time to time by the elders and the opinion leaders of that period in accordance with the demands of the particular time and place.

RIGHT TO LIFE

Article Three of the *Universal Declaration of Human Rights* declares that "Everyone has the right to life, liberty and security of person." Article Six states that "Everyone has the right to recognition everywhere as a person before law." *The International Covenant on Civil and Political Rights* (1966), Article Six, states that "Every human being has the inherent right to life." These and other declarations and affirmations raise the question: How do we define a "person," a "human being"? Who has a right to life depends upon the answer to that question.

Dr. A. Ramaswamy Iyengar, explained to me that, according to ancient *Samkhya* philosophy, there are two ultimate principles in the universe: *purusha* (soul) and *prkriti* (body). The soul is immutable (*kutastha*) and imperishable (*nitya*).[22] The soul, also called *atman*, descends into the zygote, produced from the union of the sperm and ovum, along with the mind, which carried with it the influences of major actions done in previous states of existence. "Life starts with the union of the sperm and the ovum. Individuality is reckoned from that moment. It is at the moment of the sperm-ovum union that the transmigrating *atman* (or *purusha*) gets its material encrustation, as dictated by his previous *karma*."

According to the Catholic point of view, a new human being comes into existence from the moment of conception. This is consonant with ancient Indian thought. All rights as a person accrue to the new human being and must be respected as such.

Interventions in the life and growth of the new human being should be such as to maintain and improve the quality of life. Therapeutic procedures done on the human embryo are licit, if there is respect for the life and integrity of the person (embryo/fetus). These procedures should not involve disproportionate risk, and they must be directed toward healing, improvement in health, and survival.

The child growing in the womb cannot be considered an object which can be disposed of as thought fit by the mother or any other person. What happens if an injury is caused to a fetus while in the uterus? Can damages be claimed? If the answer is yes, then the child is a person. If the fetus is a person, can the life of this individual be ended by procedures approved by others? Most doctors in India do not wish to become entangled in this debate.

ABORTION

Indian law allows abortion "if the continuance of pregnancy would involve a risk to the life of the pregnant woman or grave injury to her physical or mental health."

Abortion was a common practice in earlier times. Because it was illegal, it was performed in a clandestine manner. The passing of the law made medical termination of pregnancy legal under certain conditions, supposedly for safe-guarding the health of the mother.

Since April 1972, Indian doctors have been zealously performing abortions on demand. They advertise blatantly and invite women to have abortions done at their clinics. All of this has raised many ethical issues. The government has supported and encouraged abortions because it sees them as one more method of population control.

Although abortion is legal, many find it immoral. It is severely condemned in the *Vedic, Upanishadic*, the later *puranic* (old) and *smriti* literature. But most people in India, including physicians, do not see anything unethical or immoral in carrying out medical termination of pregnancy within the first trimester, seeing it as a contribution to the greater good of the country in light of the expanding population.

Paragraph Three of the *Code of Ethics of the Medical Council of India* says: "I will maintain the utmost respect for human life from the time of conception." There arises as a result of this moral code, a conflict between the rights of two persons, the mother and the growing fetus. Has the mother the right to destroy the life of the child she is carrying in her womb? Would that right be something akin to the possession of some material good, which can be disposed of as the mother wants, without consideration of the right of the unborn child?

The use of aborted embryos is also an ethical issue. A headline in New Delhi recently proclaimed: "Ban urged on embryo sale for brain transplants." At the World Neurological Congress in New Delhi, a physician from Holland stated that international legislation is required to prevent mothers from selling the growing embryos for transplantation of the fetal brain into the brains of patients with Parkinson's disease. According to him, "This will be a worldwide reality within a few years." A Chinese paper claimed that doctors in a Chinese hospital have successfully treated ten patients with Parkinson's disease with tissue taken from four-month-old embryos. The question is: Is it ethical for a doctor to participate in a business which encourages women to get pregnant and abort the fetus for financial considerations?

SEX PRE-SELECTION, SEX DETERMINATION, AND FEMALE FETICIDE

There are a number of methods available for sex determination and sex selection. Like many traditional practices and mores, these methods of selection are pro-male and anti-female, in that they are most often used as a basis for a decision in favor of female feticide.

It is perhaps peculiar to India that prenatal determination of sex is used as a means of rejecting a female fetus. If the test shows a female fetus, and if the parents request it, the doctor performs an abortion. Such abortion clinics thrive in the country, in spite of public opinion against the practice. Even so, many physicians continue to selectively abort female fetuses, misusing prenatal tests for sex-determination. Professional organizations such as that of the gynecologists and obstetricians in Bombay have advocated social boycott of those indulging in such unethical activities as aborting female fetuses after sex determination tests. But it is not easy, as the Secretary of the Bombay Obstetric and Gynecological Society commented, because of the difficulty in proving conclusively that such actions have been taken.

The general opinion in the country is that abortion is criminal and sinful when performed merely because the child is female. Considering the situation in our country concerning dowry, the status of women, and perennial difficulties and hardships for women and their parents, however, the practice is understandable. There are quite a few people in the Indian society who justify female feticide because of the social custom of dowry. And there are quite a few physicians who would like to take advantage of the opportunity to make quick financial gains.

The government, though proclaiming itself to be against female feticide, does not seem to be too keen to implement that policy effectively. Abortion is encouraged because it helps to control the population. India has a male/female ratio adverse to women (935 women to 1,000 men) according to the 1981 census. The availability of sex pre-selection, sex determination, and female feticide will worsen this imbalance.

INFANTICIDE

There is a growing tendency in many parts of the world toward infanticide if the newborn is diagnosed as having deformities compatible with life, but likely to put a serious burden on the family (for example, children with spina bifida). This practice occurs much less frequently in India. Parents have always accepted these children as part of their fate or *karma*. But there are a growing number of people who advocate that the choice of infanticide or nontreatment be left to the parents. These people say that if the parents feel incapable psychologically, physically, or financially to bring up a grossly abnormal child, the decision is up to them at the time of birth. To kill the child at a future date would be murder.

There are also instances where infanticide has occurred because the child was a female. It has also been the custom to do away with the newborn female child if the mother died during childbirth. But Guru Amar Dass, the third Guru of the Sikhs, opposed and condemned this practice.

In *Vedic* times, there was no reference to infanticide of children born in wedlock, but there is reference to death by exposure of the child of unmarried women.[12] Manu advised the king to order the death sentence when anyone killed a woman, a child, or a brahmana. "Neither in this world nor in the next can any action leading to the injury of living beings be productive of good results. The conduct of persons who do not perform *vratas* (religious ceremonies) but whose minds are not given to killing can lead to heaven."[19] The majority of physicians in India are completely against infanticide, even when the newborn has many defects at birth.

EUTHANASIA

India does not allow suicide or the aiding and abetting of suicide. But there have been questions raised about this position. The Law Commission in its 42nd report stated: "It is a monstrous procedure to inflict further suffering on an individual who has already found life so miserable, his chances of happiness so slender, that he has been willing to face pain and death in order to cease living."

The questions most commonly asked when discussing euthanasia have been well-formulated by Das Gupta: "Does a person not have the right to quit a life which, according to him or her, is not worth living? Is the right to die not implicit in the right to live."[4] No documents allowing euthanasia in ancient times have been found. But there were advocates among the ancient physicians for abandoning treatment when the disease had reached a stage from which recovery was considered unlikely.

According to Hindu philosophy, that which is born must die to be reborn according to individual *karma*. In Sikhism, death is not the end of life. The soul merges with the Lord, to be put into another life at His discretion. The soul is deathless and restless until it merges in the Lord.

Most people reject positive euthanasia, the bringing about of death in an active manner. There are exceptions among the intellectuals at present. Most people, however, accept suffering as part of their fate, resulting from *karma*. But there are many who favor the omission of treatment, with the intention of not prolonging the process of dying. They also favor measures to relieve constant agony, suffering, and pain, even if these measures might have a secondary effect of shortening life.

AIH/AID/SURROGATE MOTHERHOOD

The desire to have children is a dominant one, to be fulfilled if at all possible. What is to be done when there are impediments to having a child in the natural way and there is no way of overcoming sterility in one or the other partner? One solution is adoption. But many people desire to be the biological parents of their children.

What do the ancients say? According to Charaka Samhita, "The man without progeny is like a tree that yields no shade, which has no branches, which bears no fruit and is devoid of any pleasing odour."

India's social structure requires a son who is expected to provide support for his parents in old age. He is also required to perform certain religious rites on the death of the parents. A married woman is under social pressure to conceive soon after marriage. A sterile woman is considered inauspicious. There was at one time a practice called *niyoga*, or appointment of a male to have intercourse with the wife or widow of a childless person in order to conceive a son.[12] It was also the practice to appoint a widow to have intercourse with the husband to conceive a son when a couple had no children or only daughters.

There were a number of conditions necessary before *niyoga* was allowed:

1. The husband must have had no son.
2. The *gurus*, or elders, in family council, must make the decision to appoint the widow (whom they choose) to raise a male child for the husband.
3. The male person appointed to have intercourse with the wife or widow (when the husband was dead) must have been:
   (a) the husband's brother,
   (b) a *sapinda* or *sagotra* of the husband (a close relation or belonging to the same group) or a *saparivara* (a person of the same caste).
4. The person appointed and the widow must not have been motivated by lust, but only by a sense of duty.
5. The relationship was to last only until one son was born (two according to some).
6. The widow must have been comparatively young.

If the stringent conditions were not met, he or she would be punished severely. The many restrictions imposed meant that *niyoga* must not have been very prevalent.

While the ancient *dharmasastras* like Gautama allowed *niyoga*, there were other *dharmasastras* and writers, almost as old as Gautama, who condemned the practice and forbade it. Manu, for example, condemned it in the strongest terms possible. Instances of *niyoga*, rare even in ancient times, gradually became rarer as time passed. By the first centuries of the Christian era it was totally prohibited.

To whom did the child of *niyoga* belong? There was a difference of opinion. It was either (1) or (2) as follows:

1. If there was an agreement between the widow's elders and the person appointed, or between the begetter and the husband himself, that the child should belong to the husband, then the child belonged to the latter.
2. The son belonged to both the begetter and the husband of the wife.

Modern methods of artificial insemination by husband or donor and surrogate mother seem to be technological variations of this ancient procedure. The main difference is the possible commercialization in the case of surrogate motherhood. And the motives of surrogates and arrangers may be different than those of participants in the practice of *niyoga*.

In ancient times, there were no difficulties in the upbringing of the child. With the joint family system providing a close-knit community, the child was readily accepted as a member of the family.

MEDICAL EDUCATION

The process of training often determines which ethical values are held by the physician. Emphasis on medical ethics can affect the professional behavior of a future physician. In Indian medical schools today, there are few courses on ethics and related subjects. There are some exceptions, but they do not constitute even ten percent of the institutions in the country.

Concerning instructions to medical students, Charaka[10] says:

1. Your action must be free from ego, vanity, worry, agitation of mind or envy; your actions must be carefully planned, with concern for the patient and in keeping with the instructor's advice.
2. Your unceasing efforts must, at all costs (*sarvatmana*) be directed towards giving health to the suffering patient (*aturanam arogya*).
3. You must never harbor feelings of ill-will toward your patient, whatever the provocation, even if it entails risk to your life (*jivitahetor api api aturebhyo nabidrohavyam*).
4. You should never entertain thoughts (*manasapi*) of sexual misconduct or thoughts of appropriating property that does not belong to you.
5. Take no liquor, commit no sin, nor keep company with the wicked.
6. Your speech must be soft (*salakshna*) pleasant (*sarmya*), virtuous (*dhanya*), truthful (*satya*), useful (*hita*) and moderate (*mita*).
7. What you do must be appropriate to the time and the place in which you practice, and you must be mindful in whatever you do (*smriti-mata*).
8. Your efforts must be unremitting (*nityam yatnavata cha*).
9. Do not reveal to others what goes on in the patient's household (*aturakula pravarthayah*).
10. Even when you are learned and proficient, do not show off.

It is difficult to master the entirety of medical science; therefore, one must be diligent (*apramatta*) in maintaining constant contact with this branch of learning.

According to the ancients, medical wisdom is acquired by three methods (*upayani*):

1. Study (*adhyayana*), earnest and continuous.
2. Teaching (*adhyapana*), after examining the student and ascertaining his character, ability, health, and interest and imparting lessons concerning life in general, the medical profession, medical ethics, and the science of medicine.
3. Academic discussions (*tatvidya-sambhasha*) with colleagues and fellow students to enrich one's own knowledge, to obtain clarity of knowledge and get rid of doubts, to deepen one's understanding and learn new methods and ideas, and to become skilled in expressing one's thoughts.

Note that active learning is placed before teaching and that there is a specific mention of medical ethics among the broad subdivisions to be taught.

At the time of initiation, the student had to take an oath. But what was more interesting was that the teacher also had to take an oath: "When you, on your part, keep your vows and if I do not respond fully and impart all my knowledge, I shall become a sinner and my knowledge shall go fruitless."[12]

The major problem that has arisen in India recently is the admission of students into "Capitation Fee Medical Colleges" based on the payment of a large sum by the student (or parent), usually Rs.300,000 to Rs.400,000. Such payments are sometimes not recorded. Other students, even though they may be far more qualified academically and otherwise, are not admitted because they cannot afford to pay the large "fee." Since the basis for admission is the ability to pay such a large amount, many unethical practices arise. The whole environment becomes commercialized and vitiated; teaching and patient care are also affected.

ORGAN TRANSPLANTS

There is a big demand for organ donors, especially for kidneys. These demands and the means of meeting them are often responsible for ethical nightmares because of unscrupulous activities relating to procurement and allocation. A small proportion of kidney transplants are done with close relatives as donors. This is possible because of strong family ties. But a large majority of donors are unrelated and the kidneys are obtained commercially.

A British urologist, Dr. Michael Vurvick, discovered that wealthy Indian patients had been paying their poorer fellow countrymen to be donors. He wrote a scathing article about Indian surgeons and their unethical practices. But this has also been occurring in other countries such as the Philippines, Turkey, and others, in which poor people are given unfair inducements of money for "donation" of kidneys. Turks have even been clandestinely brought to Britain to supply organs for British nationals.

When transplant surgery became common, doctors in India saw a potential goldmine in this procedure. There were unlimited numbers of kidney patients from the rich Middle East, in addition to wealthy Indian patients. They were prepared to pay whatever was asked. As a result, kidney transplants became a commercial proposition. A new class of agents or organ-procurers rose up. The doctors involved were not bothered about the ethical issues of stealing a kidney from an unsuspecting person. A few doctors, including Dr. B.N. Colabawala, a urologist, objected: "The trafficking that is taking place in kidneys is ethically unacceptable, morally wrong and sociologically degrading."

An estimated 100 kidney transplants involving foreign patients are performed every month in India, mostly in Bombay. Fees of Rs.50,000 or more are charged. The donors get a small portion; the agents are also paid. Those foreigners (mainly from the Middle East) who wish to obtain a kidney at a relatively cheap price make a beeline for Bombay.

It is not only illiterate people from the slums of Bombay that "donate" kidneys. Knowledgeable persons are also prepared to give up one kidney because they are in desperate need of money. A young lady working as a typist in Bangalore wrote me a pathetic letter: "I am prepared to give (up) my kidney for Rs.20,000, as I need the money to pay for the dowry of my elder sister."

The people involved in kidney trafficking will go to any lengths, without concern for the consequences. *The Times of India* (Bombay, 20 October 1989) ran the following item: "A 35 year old woman from Kashmir narrowly escaped receiving the kidney of an AIDS carrier. The transplant operation had been scheduled for tomorrow." The man who offered to give up a kidney for Rs.25,000 is a professional blood donor--and an AIDS carrier. The donor had chosen to sell one kidney since he needed the money, due to the fact that he could not get employment since he was HIV positive.

In India, almost all kidney transplants are from live donors. There have been very few cadaveric transplants. It is notable that the legality of this procedure is seriously questionable. *The Times of India* (Bombay, 18 June 1989) stated: "All kidney transplants in India are at present illegal. There is no specific law which allows a doctor to take a healthy organ from a human being for a reason which is not beneficial to the donor's health."

TERMINALLY ILL

Physicians have been brought up to preserve life and to prevent death. The ancient teaching has been that awareness of the incurability of a patient's disease should not cause the physician to withdraw care or treatment. As long as the patient breathes, it is the duty of the physician to provide treatment (*tatvat pratikriya karya yavae chvasiti manavah*).[16] But there is also another view: One should know when to stop treatment. Among the qualities that brought credit to a physician was the withdrawal of treatment from a patient whose condition was definitely moribund (*upekshanam prakristheshu*).[10] The two apparently contradictory dictums probably mean that heroic treatment was to be withdrawn and only care given to the terminally ill in order to reduce suffering.

Current medical opinion is also in line with the above. Prolonging life with the help of machines when there is no chance of recovery or in patients suffering great pain and distress because of incurable illness has been questioned more frequently in recent times. If restoration of health is no longer possible and death is imminent, the physician need not do anything extraordinary or heroic to prolong living or dying, but it is proper and necessary to relieve pain and suffering. These measures have to be taken, even if they may incidently shorten life. The physician is expected to assist the patient in achieving a peaceful death.

TO TELL OR NOT TO TELL

According to Charaka and other physicians of the ancient days, a doctor must be careful when telling the patient that his or her illness may be incurable.

Charaka advises that it should not be told bluntly, for it may shock the patient. Preferably, this information is made known to the patient's relatives, and even to state officials to protect the doctor from prosecution should the patient die under his care. Treatment of a heroic nature is to be undertaken only with the consent of the relatives and elders.

Today, doctors differ in their opinions concerning how much information to provide and when to tell the truth to their patients who are dying. The many conflicting considerations include the patient's right to know, the benefit to the patient, and possible harm.

A study conducted in the Postgraduate Institute of Medical Education and Research, Chandigarh, showed that 69.2 percent of doctors favored telling the truth, while 30.8 percent did not believe in telling the truth to terminally ill patients.[11] Most physicians favored involvement of family members and close relatives. In view of the family structure and the closer ties among relatives in Indian society, this aspect is of obvious importance.

CONCLUSION

We have moved a long way from the precepts and practices of the ancients. The changes have affected ethics in general, as well as those of the medical profession. Part of the shift has occurred as a result of the values cherished in ancient times; part of it is due to different ways of thinking, influenced to some extent by contact with other cultures; and part of it has resulted from the advances in science and technology. The result is that we are in a state of confusion. We have been creating situations in which our ethical responses have been slow to develop, or even nonexistent. What is the solution to the dilemmas with which we are faced? Perhaps the answer is a judicious blending of the ancient with the modern. Such an integrated approach will hopefully elicit responses which may be made progressively relevant to the times and needs while still based on the cherished ideals of human relationships.

NOTES

1   Bhattacharya N.L., ed. *Susruta Samhita*. Mysore: University of Mysore, 1973.

2   Chren M.M., Landfeld C., Seth M., Thomas H. Doctors, drug companies and gifts. *JAMA*--India, 1990;6:641-644.

3   D'Silva J. *Newstimes* (Hyderabad) October 22, 1989.

4   Das Gupta S.M. Mercy killing, an analysis based on human rights. *Proceedings of the International Conference on Health Policy Ethics and Human Values*. New Delhi: 1986.

5   Duggal R. Exploding the population bomb myth. *Medico-Friends Circle Bulletin*, 1989;152-153.

6   Goldsmith Marsha F. Oregon pioneers "more ethical" medicaid coverage with priority setting project. *JAMA* 1989;262:176-7.

7   Haring B. *Medical Ethics*. St. Paul Publications, 1972.

8   Holder A.R. *Medical Malpractice Law*. New York: John Wiley and Sons, 1975.

9   *ICSSR-ICMR Study on Health for All--An Alternative Strategy*. Pune: Indian Institute of Education, 1981.

10   Jayadeva V., ed. *Charaka Samhita*. Delhi: Motilal Benarsidass, 1986.

11   Jindal S.K., Jindal U.N. To tell or not to tell: professional practices in the case of dying. *Proceedings of the International Conference on Health Policy: Ethics and Human Values*. New Delhi: 1986.

12   Kane P.V. *History of Dharmasastras*. 2nd ed, Pune: Bhandarkar Oriental Research Institute, 1974.

13   McCarthy Donald G., Moraczewski A. *Moral Responsibility in Prolonging Life Decisions*. St. Louis:Pope John Centre, 1981.

14   Palmer P.E.S. The epidemic of investigations, *International Journal of Epidemiology*, 1985;14:359-365.

15   Radhakrishnan S. *Indian Philosophy*. Delhi: Oxford University Press, 1929.

16   Ramachandra R~o, ed. *Encyclopaedia of Indian Medicine*, Bombay:Popular Book Prakashan, 1987.

17   Ramachandran C.K. The total life-vision in ancient Indian Medicine. *Ancient Science of Life* 1986;5:139-42.

18   Ramalingaswamy V. Another revolution in Medicine, Keynote address, International Seminar on Recent Trends in Non-invasive Organ Imaging, 1986.

19   Sarkar B.K. *Indian Culture*, Patna:IB Corporation, 1936.

20   Srinivasamurthy R., Somnath Chatter ji, Sriram T.G., Parvatha Vardhini, Mamatha Shetty, and Raghavan K.S. Informed consent for drug trials:a systematic study. *NIMHANS Journal* 1988;6:145-9.

21   Thairu K., Manufacturers and users in joint endeavour, World Health Forum, 1989;10:23.

22   Wadhwani Y.K. Subtle bodies postulated in the classical Samkhya system. *Journal of the L.D. Institute of Indology*, 1976;5:29-40.

14

The Interaction Between Thai Traditional and Western Medicine in Thailand

Attajinda Deepadung

INTRODUCTION

The main objective of this paper is to present an overview of Thai traditional medical systems and their interaction with Western counterparts. My contention is that the health behavior of the traditional Thai is a rational response to his or her perception of the causes of illnesses. By viewing these perceptions as rational, we can get an insight into the structure and dynamics of Thai health behavior. Consequently, I will emphasize the conceptual elements that underlie all aspects of traditional Thai medical systems. I will also make an attempt to show that the Western world has its own culture-specific medical systems which provide an obvious and striking contrast to the traditional Thai medical systems. Since the metaphysical and epistemological foundations are noticeably different, attempts to integrate the two systems would encounter unresolvable difficulties. Therefore, I recommend that we support both systems in the hope that they can co-exist and compliment each other.

THAI TRADITIONAL MEDICINE

Disease, with its pain and suffering, is the most predictable of human conditions; it is a biological as well as a cultural universal. In response to such a threat, people, as cultural beings, have, over time, developed social institutions, etiological theories, and therapeutic techniques to enable them to cope with the dislocations occasioned by illness-induced disabilities. The Thai people are no exception. They have learned to employ adaptive strategies in response to the threats posed by diseases. These strategies can be perceived in the Thai social and cultural traditions that have evolved in order to enhance health.

In the face of disease, the Thai have developed a vast complex of knowledge, beliefs, techniques, roles, norms, values, ideologies, attitudes, customs, rituals, and symbols that interlock to form a mutually reinforcing and supporting system.[13] This vast complex constitutes the Thai traditional medical system. As this definition indicates, Thai traditional medicine embraces the totality of health knowledge, beliefs, skills, and practices of people from all walks of life. Therefore, the term is used in a comprehensive sense to include all clinical and nonclinical activities, formal and informal institutions, and any other activities that, however tangentially, bear on the health levels of the group and promote the optimum functioning of society.

To put it in different terms, Thai traditional medicine embraces all the beliefs, practices, and local wisdom which are the product of indigenous cultural development. The primary purpose of this system is to raise the level of health and to reduce the incidence of threats to health. Thai traditional medical systems, in other words, are integral parts of total cultural patterns. Pellegrino caught the spirit of this claim and wrote, "Every culture has developed a system of medicine which bears an indissoluble and reciprocal relationship to the prevailing worldview. The medical behavior of individuals and groups is incomprehensible apart from general cultural history."[9]

In Thailand, to understand the traditional Thai medical system, one cannot overlook three essential ingredients which are fundamental components of Thai culture: (1) the belief in supernatural deities, (2) the influence of Brahmanism, and (3) Buddhism.

Komart Chugsatiensap, in *The Thai Medical System in the Rural Area*, classifies Thai traditional medicine into four major categories: (1) empirical medicine, (2) supernatural medicine, (3) astrological medicine, and (4) humoral medicine.

Empirical Medicine

Obviously, the causes of illnesses have been of interest to mankind for a long time. Although human curiosity has played a part in motivating investigation, a more important reason for research has been the need to ascertain causes of illnesses so that preventive measures may be found and treatments developed. Accepted treatments for illness in empirical medicine were not limited, of course, to the more complicated therapies used for chronic debilitating diseases. Procedures and prescriptions were also devised for handling everyday conditions.

In Thai culture, there were individuals who developed skills needed to provide particular forms of treatment such as setting bones, midwifery, and preparing herbs to be given for specific symptoms. Once a successful procedure was discovered it was incorporated into the culture and passed on from generation to generation.

As part of their regional culture, the Thai sought out ways of treating threatening diseases (always within their own setting). Based on different conceptual understandings, diseases were given different names. Chuengsatiensap[4] classifies Thai medicine in three categories: Folk Medicine, Individual Treatment, and Local Healer.

Folk Medicine

Thai villagers can be said to be traditional pharmacists who administer specific herbs and mixtures of herbs for specific, local, but common illnesses. Medicinal plants are locally grown and easily accessible. For example, a mixture of dried custard apple and limewater, neutralized by turmeric, was used to treat abscesses, and sap from the ebony family was used as a laxative.

Individual Treatment

In each culture, sparked by the desire to cope with illness, people try to conform to certain behavioral patterns in order to achieve health. In rural Thailand, particularly in the northern region, there is a variety of traditional taboos. Most taboos are a part of the local culture and are elements of learned behavior, acquired partly by deliberate instruction on the part of parents and partly through observation of the behavior of relatives and other members of the community.

There are many customs relating to childbirth. Rauyajin[11] found that the "roasting" custom is believed by a great number of rural villagers to be crucial for the postpartum mother. It is thought that, during this practice, the heat from the charcoal helps involute the uterus and that mothers who do not "roast" will experience poor and failing health when they are older.

It is also a local custom that the postpartum mother should stop eating ordinary food and have only rice and salt. The consumption of beef and certain kinds of vegetables, fish, and eggs is strictly forbidden during pregnancy because it is believed to endanger the pregnant woman's health and bring about difficulties in childbirth. In the south of the northern Thailand region, inclusion in the diet of certain food items, such as eels, is encouraged for easy delivery. Chicken, morning glory, and Thai spinach are believed to help increase the mother's milk during the breastfeeding period. Villagers in Ayuddhaya hold the view that fermented food, ice, and fruits such as guava and jackfruit are to be forbidden during pregnancy.

Although a variety of health-related dietary norms exist, the basic conventional wisdom of the Thai about food, as noted in the preceding paragraph, is marked by major gaps in their understanding of nutrition. Perhaps the most important of these gaps is the frequent failure to recognize a general relationship between diet and the maintenance of health. Consequently, malnutrition exists because eating habits reflect a whole complex of culinary activities, likes and dislikes, folk wisdom, beliefs, taboos, and superstitions associated with the production, preparation, and consumption of food.

Local Healers

Local healers generally have inherited a working knowledge of traditional medicine from their ancestors. They are responsible for the treatment of special, localized, and complex diseases. Relying mainly on knowledge gained from experience, they practice without having been trained in any of the systematic methods of modern medicine. These healers can be classified roughly into five groups.

1. Herbalists (who treat by boiling, or by rubbing in herbs)
2. Bonesetters
3. Midwives
4. Masseurs
5. Specialists (who treat particular medical problems such as hemorrhoids, snake bite, rabies).

Supernatural Medicine

It seems clear that rational beings have constantly aspired to make the most comprehensive and fundamental inquiries into the nature of what there is in the world and why certain things happen within societies or to individuals as members of a society. The question "What brought that about?" is a necessary question, one which we cannot reasonably refuse to ask. But the answer to such questions is limited to that which can be sought either within or beyond experience. Different people provide different answers. The Thai maintain that there must be a supersensible "Being of beings," a necessary Being entirely different from the contingent things with which we are familiar, a Being who lies beyond the range of the senses but whose powers could bring about either health and social stability or disruption of the whole. In attempting to protect themselves from these threats, people have sought solutions to problems of illness within a framework of beliefs in a supernatural power.

Recommended treatments are, of course, directed at requiring or prohibiting behavior which is known or believed to be causally connected to health conditions. When people believe that illness is caused by angry gods or resentful ancestors who are punishing sin, "the obvious procedure to prevent it is confession or, even better, the meticulous observation of social taboos and the careful execution of rites and ceremonies owed to the gods and the ancestors."[1]

In all parts of Thailand, rural areas in particular, the Thai live in a theoretical universe of complex causality involving human agents, their souls, and "supernatural" entities and forces. Human diseases are thought to be caused principally by supernatural entities and forces that may have an evil intent when interacting with humans. The names of these deities, which are different in different localities, all begin with "Phi," which means "Spirit." Some of these are: Phi phaya than, Phi puta, Phi chue, Phi pa, Phi dong, and Phi nam in the northeast.

These spirits are thought to be responsible for the modification of human environment. Just as in current Western scientific thought, where the environment is believed to be conditioned by chemical and physical processes and where those same notions are extended to an understanding of the functioning of the human organism, people in ancient Thailand applied their beliefs about the action of spirits (demons) and gods to their understanding of human illness and health. Since it was believed that they lived in a continuous battle with a great number of spirits who might inflict bodily and mental damage on them, behavior for preventive and curative purposes became, for the Thai, a logical application of their understanding of the nature of things. Where gods were believed to cause diseases as punishments for prior misdeeds, a particular lifestyle was identified and advocated as necessary to avoid such retributions. As a result, instructions about how to act in order to prevent illness and cure diseases became functionally related to a commonly accepted worldview.

In other words, one should not be surprised that Thai ideas about living harmoniously in one's natural environment reappeared in their prescriptions for structuring an ideal society. The worldview of members of a society shows a remarkable congruence between their concept of physiological health and their concept of social order. Phi puta, a spirit reputed to live in northeastern Thailand, is highly regarded as a lawgiver and creator of social order. It is therefore quite a common sight to see a spirit house built at the entrance to each village in this region. Tao chum, individuals who perceive themselves and are perceived by their communities as the mediums for these causative and creative powers, are said to be able to communicate with Phi puta.

Phi chau act as protectors of the family and are specifically in charge of general well-being and harmony. In cases of misconduct, (a quarrel between husband and wife, adultery, or abandonment of a family), Phai chau might inflict bodily or mental damage or cause disasters of various sorts. In some cases, injuries might occur to other members of the family and not to the culprit. Such harms are believed to be punishment for a prior misdeed or a particular lifestyle which needs to be avoided. Various kinds of protectors exist in different regions of the country. These protectors include Phi or spirits, and different sacred objects dedicated to asking mercy of Lord Buddha.

In certain regions of the country, there is widespread belief in a hierarchy among the spirits. In general, Phi fa (or the spirit of the sky) is regarded as the most important. To communicate with Phi fa, one has to use a medium to perform certain rituals in order to ask for forgiveness and the restoration of health. The treatment or healing ceremony usually involves the following three crucial steps:

1. A diagnostic dance is performed to find out what actually went wrong and who caused the illnesses.
2. A treatment dance is performed to heal the sickness by asking for forgiveness, offering favorite items, or even sacrificing animals. Repeat performances

may be done in cases where there has been serious wrongdoing or misconduct.
3. A farewell dance is performed after the patient is fully recovered in order
to express gratitude.

Chuengsatiensap indicates in his findings that in diagnostic dances, the words
used concentrate on social misconduct or disruption.[3] A patient is thought to
have violated the village code of ethics and thus contributed directly to the
illness. Examples of violation of the code of ethics include: a wife quarreling with
her husband, a person cutting down a tree without permission from Phi, children
abusing their elders, people engaging in such selfish or undesirable behavior as
the blocking of an irrigation canal.

Shamanism

Another form of supernatural medicine that developed in the face of
diseases is the healing practice called "shamanism." This technique is used to
improve a person's *karma* or "destiny." The doctrine of *karma* is believed by the
Thai to be very significant in promoting health or causing disease. Illnesses might
be caused by the sins or shortcomings of a previous existence, while longevity is
believed to be largely due to *karma*. Although the doctrine focuses on the inner
acceptance of disease and gives a ready-made explanation of its cause, nowhere
is a man advised to submit to illness without attempting a cure. Since the evil
brought about by *karma* cannot be estimated with certainty, and the harmful
effects of sins can be offset by merit gained from performing good deeds, there
is every reason for a sick person to seek all the medical help possible in order to
achieve health.

Karma is generally thought to be the source of congenital defects. A man
born with a deformed hand, for example, is believed to have incurred this
misfortune as a result of an evil deed (for instance striking a father or a mother)
done by the same hand in a previous life. This, again, does not preclude attempts
at improving one's condition by surgery, since the duration of the karmatic
punishment is not known and the trouble might be only temporary. Puntong
states that "practitioners (shamans) are vehicles of those deities who are
directed towards the healing of human suffering."[10] When a patient comes to see
the shaman, the healer will first diagnose whether the ailment is physical,
psychosomatic, spirit inflicted, or the result of magic. Then the shaman treats it
accordingly. For physical illness, the treatment usually consists of local herbs,
massages, stream baths, or blessed water, accompanied by some healing rituals.

In brief, such medical beliefs and practices are invoked in order to explain
all misfortunes and to control the social environment. The culture tells its
members how to conduct their lives--what work to do, where to live, who to
marry, what to worship, and so on. A society thus prescribes and allocates roles
of responsibility for the conditions of oneself and others. While a society's

members, for various reasons, will not always conform to their own rules, at least some conformity to codes of behavior is likely. In this context, responsibility for disease will be distributed in various ways. Pathogens, in human and other carriers, must be contained by those who can prevent their spread. Society tells its members how healers achieve their powers, how they should use these powers, and how patients and their associates ought to behave. While the prescribed behavior may not, in fact, produce the healing it is supposed to bring about, it may satisfy the member's expectations about proper healing methods. Society and its culture thus prescribe a system of therapy based on belief and custom.

Astrological Medicine

In considering the Thai traditional medical systems, we cannot overlook the significance of astrology and its impact on Thai society. Most Thai still hold the view that the heavenly bodies determine human characteristics and the course of human affairs, including illnesses. The movement of these heavenly bodies, it is believed, will have an impact on one's life. Astrologers are thought to have a correct understanding of the influence of planets and stars on earthly affairs and to be able to predict or affect the destinies of individuals, groups, or nations. They often act as fortune tellers as well as healers.

The treatment usually commences with an astrologer making a diagnosis based on astrology. His work consists mainly of making a determination as to which heavenly bodies are having an influence on a patient at a particular time. If the illnesses are caused by bad luck, astrologers provide suggestions and instructions about how this bad luck might be driven out. Certain rituals and ceremonies (such as floating kratong of misfortune in a river) are likely to follow. The success of these rituals depends largely on the patient's luck.

Humoral Medicine

Humoral medicine is a naturalistic system which explains illness in terms of an equilibrium model. Health occurs when all the basic body elements (the humors, the yin/yang, and the ayurvedic *dosha*) are in a balance appropriate to the age and condition of the individual. When this balance is upset from without or within by natural forces such as heat or cold, or sometimes by strong emotions, illness follows. Historically speaking, humoral medicine has its roots in the West in the Greek theory of the four elements (earth, water, air, and fire) widely recognized in the sixth century BC. By the time of Hippocrates (born about 460 BC), this theory had been augmented by the parallel concept of the four qualities--hot, cold, dry, moist. When integrated with the original theory, it produced the concept of the four humors with their associated qualities: blood (hot and moist), phlegm (cold and moist), black bile, also called "melancholy" (cold and dry), and yellow bile, or "choler" (hot and dry). That this equilibrium theory of health was further developed in ancient Greece is evidenced by Hippocrates' description of disease. "The human body contains blood, phlegm, yellow bile, and black bile. These are the things that make up its constitution and cause its pain and health. Health is primarily that state in which these constituent substances are in the correct proportion to each other, both in strength and quantity, and are well mixed."[3]

The four humors, writes Hippocrates, "have specific and different names because there are essential differences in their appearance. . . . They are dissimilar in their qualities of heat, cold, dryness, and moisture."[3] Greek humoral medicine was brought to the East and to the West as seen in the histories of medicine in Persia, Pakistan, and other Southwestern Asian countries. The basic classical Greek medical beliefs began, at some point, to influence almost all traditional medical systems.

The *ayurvedic* theory of medicine also claims that the universe is composed of the four elements recognized by the Greeks (earth, water, fire, air), plus a fifth--ether. The structured arrangement of these elements is the body, a microcosm of the universe, in which each of the elements possesses five "subtle" and five "material" forms. The human body also has three humors, or *dosha* (hence the "tridosha" theory): phlegm, or mucus; bile, or gall; and wind, or flatulence. Good health exists when the three dosha are in equilibrium; ill health manifests itself when one or more of the *dosha* are not functioning properly (Leslie 1969; Opler 1963). The *dosha* also are associated with age and the seasons: phlegm with youth and the growing season, bile with middle age and the rainy season, and wind with old age and cold and dry weather.[2]

The central concept of Chinese cosmology is that there are "dual forces of yin and yang, where continuous interaction lies behind all natural phenomena, including the constitution and functioning of the human body."[2] This concept occurs in traditional Chinese medicine where the proper balance within the body of yin and yang is essential and vital for good heath. "This principle of harmony, which views disease as essentially due to its impairment through external or internal physical or mental causes, has remained central to all of later Chinese medicine."[5]

Chinese philosophers and physicians recognized that the five elements of water, fire, metal, wood, and earth were all contained in the human body and all linked to physiological processes and to specific internal organs. The number five was, in fact, the basis of an elaborate system of numerical concordancy in which most phenomena were thought to occur in sets of five: seasons, directions, musical notes, colors, emotions, bodily orifices, food flavors, internal organs. Other instances were found in the agreement of the number of days of the year with the 365 drugs of the earliest surviving pharmacopoeia[5] and the 368 bodily surface points recognized for insertion of acupuncture needles.[16] The preoccupation with philosophical elegance unquestionably hindered medical advances which might have occurred with greater attention to empirical observations and experimentation.

In humoral medicine, Thai healers simplified ayurvedic medicine by practicing it as locally adapted and, for hundreds of years, they made use of some forms of Chinese medicine. The main body of medical knowledge was probably introduced from India at the same time as Buddhism. Notable is the complete absence of surgery. Herbs were used exclusively for treatment.

It should be noted that Thai traditional healers do not exhibit an eager interest in money. Western physicians, however, are characterized as greedy. They are compared unfavorably to their primitive counterparts who, it is assumed, have had greater concern for the welfare of humanity. Like most stereotypes, this one is far from true. In all societies, healers receive compensation in some form; Thai traditional healers also receive compensation. The kinds and amounts of payment vary greatly, of course, depending on factors such as the length and cost of the healer's professional training, as well as the extent to which power is said to stem from the "grace" of a deity. Among herbalists, the cost of treatment is whatever the patient wishes to leave. In some cases, patients are able to pay only a very small amount, not in return for treatment but out of respect for the healer's honored teachers.

In brief, such medical beliefs and practices are invoked in order to explain all misfortunes and to control the social environment. The culture tells its members how to conduct their lives--what work to do, where to live, who to marry, what to worship, and so on. A society thus prescribes and allocates roles of responsibility so that conditions of healthy living may be experienced by all of its members. While a society's members, for various reasons, will not always conform to their own laws, at least some conformity to the rules of behavior is likely. Accordingly, the culture will be responsible in various ways for disease. Cultural practices, including conformity to the rules, will be at least partly responsible for the spread and prevention of disease. Because it is a major influence in the thinking of those who allocate physical and social resources, a society's culture will also be a significant factor in the distribution of physical and social sources of healing. It will tell members how healers achieve the powers they have, how they should use these powers, and how patients and their associates should behave. While the prescribed behavior may not in fact produce the healing it is supposed to provide, it nevertheless may conform to the members' beliefs about proper healing. Culture thus describes and prescribes a system of therapy.

To sum up, in Thailand the practice of medicine exists in two distinct forms, that of Western medicine and that of traditional medicine. Physicians of Western medicine are educated primarily in European and American schools. This results in a very highly developed and progressive Western medical system in Thailand, the standards of which are equal to those of any country in the world.

COMMENTS

Thai traditional medical systems have been shaped, in part at least, by the presence of holistic worldviews, by the acceptance of different metaphysical beliefs regarding the nature of truth and reality, and by efforts of rural Thai to peacefully promote or, sometimes, to forcefully assure adherence to the laws inherent in their ideologies and systems. With these efforts came an acknowledgement of and support for specific conceptual medical systems as the basis of orthodox health care. Thai traditional medicine is not one single conceptual medical system but a combination of Indian, Buddhist, and Chinese medical traditions combined with local wisdom. All these components help to form Thai culture as well as its traditional medical systems. Such effects on the culture also specify the nosology, etiology, and theories of healing, dividing them as to conditions of health and disease, probable causes of such states, and means of their alteration. More broadly, Thai culture defines the divisions of things and the workings of causal and other forces in the universe. Causes may be seen as located within persons, in relations between persons, or in "natural" or "supernatural" entities or forces. Thus, individuals may be regarded as wholly responsible, partly responsible, or not responsible at all, (ie., as "patients" or as bearers of affliction) for their disease states and/or their health; similarly, healers may be regarded as wholly responsible, partly responsible, or only vehicles of greater forces in healing.

Such differences in conception of and beliefs relating to causes and effects greatly influence the course of the therapeutic outlook. Patients may seek different sources of healing, largely depending on their fundamental beliefs. They will seek those competent to work within their own cultural systems and contexts. They will rationally, logically, and consistently follow the premises on which Thai culture is based.

The recommendations of healers working from the Thai traditional system of medicine was one of the most effective devised in antiquity. It was more or less closed, as far as its theory went, but it was always open to new ideas for practical therapeutic methods. Thus, Thai traditional medicine has survived to the present and still plays a significant role in healing practices. With the support of the government, Thai traditional healers are now trained in a special college where, to some extent, they learn physiology as a science as well as traditional medicine. Thus they provide an alternative medical service which is effective in the curing of many diseases and which is appreciably cheaper than Western medicine. In the process of adapting itself to the modern international system of medicine, however, the system is beginning to lose its identity.

Positive Aspects of Thai Traditional Medicine

The strengths of the Thai medical system can be considered as part of the categories of psychosocial support therapies and clinical or therapeutic activities. This is especially true of the maintenance of herbal pharmacopoeias. Many findings by anthropologists concerned with these questions indicate that it is in the category of psychosocial support therapies, and not in their category of clinical activities, that Thai traditional medicine has proven most effective. This is probably due to the fact that, to a far greater extent than in Western medicine, illness in traditional societies represents dysfunction not only within the patient's body, but also in his or her relationships with society. In addition, it may represent dysfunction within the society itself.

This view is nowhere more clearly seen than among the northern and northeastern Thai. Their conception of health is very different from ours. For them, health is symptomatic of a correct relationship between humans and their environment, which includes the supernatural environment, all kinds of Phi, the surrounding world, and other human beings. Health is associated with good psychological, physiological, and social conditions, all of which are positively valued in life. Illness, on the other hand, bears evidence that one may lose this delicate balance. It is this comprehensive human-environment context, according to which so many Thai people view illness, that explains why the role of the powerful curer (the shaman, spiritual healer, mediator, astrologer) is conceived to be far broader than that of his Western counterpart. The healer usually is not a simple therapist, one skilled in the ways of treating symptoms; indeed, he works to restore and maintain harmony between individuals, their society, and their environment. For example, Nakhon Ratchasima and Chiangmai describe the ways in which shamans, through their supernatural contacts with "deities," work to prevent illness by controlling and limiting the places and times where the villagers may cut down trees, thus avoiding undue stress on a delicately balanced ecological system. I have seen, too, how the northeastern native healer is a social and legal arbiter who, reminding his fellows of the risk of illness from social nonconformity, is able to mediate and compromise social strains that might otherwise produce major community dysfunction.

This fundamental contrast in views about the context of illness between Thai traditional medicine and Western medicine helps to explain the importance of frequent public healing ceremonies found only among Thai traditional peoples. In Rachaburi, the role of the healer resembles the role of the observer, that is, the healer appears to be an interested or amused spectator who enjoys a good show. Perhaps relatives or friends more often play active parts in rituals. For example, among the Mon family members in Rachaburi who have brought a "mediator or dancer" to conduct a healing rite for an ill member of the group, all remain during the entire ceremony, which may last up to three days. "Relatives and friends come to the ceremony and take part in the chants and prayers directed by the medicine woman and her assistant."[15] They too receive positive benefits by association from the healing, and the presence of family and friends is reassuring to the patient who feels they are all working to restore his or her health. The extent of community commitment to therapy is indicated by Vajanarat's 1972 study. He noted that Mon villagers devote about one-quarter of their time to such ceremonials.

It seems clear that Thai traditional medical systems emphasize spiritual healing. They may be founded on mistaken theories of the etiology of disease, but I see in them two striking advantages over reliance upon scientific treatments.

First, the patient is not exposed to the undesirable side effects of many of the newest drugs; herbs are less likely to upset the body balance. Second, Thai medical systems, in most cases, require the participation or presence of other persons or family members in addition to the patient, and thus help to revitalize the patient. In some cases, the family presence helps to reintegrate the patient into the community from which he has become estranged due to a misdeed or the violation of a taboo.

Another therapeutic technique is public confession (such as is required for cutting down trees). This practice reflects the extent to which the actions of a patient are believed to have endangered not only the patient but also society. In addition to providing emotional catharsis and a return of peacefulness, confession often provides relief from the burden of painful experiences.[14] To put it somewhat differently, Thai traditional medicine has a psychosocial support dimension. The healing ceremonies, in which the people have so much faith, have a psychotherapeutic effect on the patient. There is also good evidence that sprinkling of water on patients and the body massage used in some ceremonies may act as physiotherapy.

As regards the northern and northeastern Thai, traditional beliefs and practices are useful since they do what they are expected to do. From a social point of view, these beliefs and practices are necessary and even morally imperative because they are socially approved ways of dealing with disruptive and anomalous events which cannot be allowed to persist. (Adultery, cutting tall trees, and abusing elders damage the social as well as the ecological system as a whole.) From a cognitive point of view, the practices are meaningful since they communicate important ideas about the real world, and through medical praxis, they provide the means for confirming and preserving this sense of reality.

On balance, when considered not only in terms of therapeutic ends but also as regards all religious, legal, social, and psychological functions they may be expected to fulfill, I hold the view that Thai traditional systems come out remarkably well as adaptive cultural institutions which promote the well-being of Thai society as a whole.

Moreover, traditional Thai medical systems focus as a whole on the functional interrelationships of all aspects of a culture. In modern Western medicine, the emphasis is more on the distinct parts of the body. However, traditional Thai medicine is closely knit with all other cultural and social ties. It is a functional, purposeful association, in very much the same sense that an automobile engine is a purposeful association of discrete parts, a dynamic system. The units are integrated one with another so that there is logic, coherence, and pattern in the total assemblage.

Negative Aspects of Thai Traditional Systems

When we turn to the specifically clinical aspects of Thai traditional medicine, we find a wide range of responses regarding its effectiveness. The first response is an acknowledgment that herbs, barks, and roots used by traditional healers may have objective medical value. Even today the science of pharmacology is heavily indebted to herbal medicine which brings to it a storehouse of empirical knowledge. Embedded in a variegated body of healing techniques, procedures, and beliefs are many types of practical approaches, comparative tests, and treatments effective for the restoration and maintenance of human well-being. "The remarkable success of our species is due in no small part to the local solution of medical problems."[8] In response to these strongly positive evaluations, Professor Ouay Ketusinh has pointed out four negative aspects of Thai medical systems, based on humoral theory. He claims that:

1. Thai medical texts are inconsistent and vague. These factors might be due to the desire to keep ingredients secret. As a result, the texts are, to some extent, unreliable.
2. The Thai medical system lacks basic knowledge of anatomy, physiology, and pathology.
3. Thai therapeutic and diagnostic techniques are not acceptable within the biomedical model.
4. Thai traditional medicine has a strong focus on internal medicine but it lacks the practice of surgery and knowledge relevant to gynecology.

Above all, traditional medical systems, it is claimed, fail to satisfy the "disease oriented Western medical model," and therefore there is no place for them in the Western hospital. In 1934, the use of Thai medicine came to an end in Western hospitals after fifteen years of attempting to offer both practices in a Western setting.

Professor Dr. Sud Saengvichian accurately reports that the main factor leading to the discontinuation of the Thai medical system is the fact that its healers were not able to work in Western hospitals. Each individual practitioner had his or her own medical ingredients and gave out different prescriptions. Thai medical healers do not have systematic methods of treatment. Their texts are also limited in number, and teaching is done through memorization only.

After 1923, Thai medical systems were ignored by Western-trained scholars. The government had passed a medical act classifying Thai medical practitioners as "those who practice by mere experience and therefore fail to satisfy the scientific criteria for knowledge." Since then, traditional healers have found themselves on a steady, downhill run, and many have begun to look around for some other profitable occupation.

To my mind, traditional uses of such remedies evolved through a long history of trial and error--in short, through human experimentation. The methods of investigation employed by traditional herbalists are not qualitatively different from those employed in modern clinical chemotherapeutic investigations. The difference is principally a matter of time, "primitive herbalists" requiring decades or generations of testing. A line of herbalists over several generations reaches a decision based on decades of experience in treating individuals with certain illnesses; his controls are patients with similar disorders who are treated with other remedies or not treated at all. For medical practitioners, in what we have called "naturalistic" systems, this is possible. After all, classical humoral pathology, ayurvedic medicine, and traditional Chinese medicine represent a literate tradition, and at least some practitioners could read and write and therefore keep records. However, I feel that this is not a valid assumption as far as practitioners of "personalistic" medicine are concerned. Particularly in Thai society, where illiteracy is widespread, a practitioner usually learns by memorization. Some of the Thai basic texts are written in poetic form to facilitate memorization. Moreover, Thai practitioners lack the means of keeping records and they lack comprehension of the notion of controls and of statistical inference, both of which are essential to an empirical approach.

I see a fundamental dichotomy in the Thai traditional medical systems and scientific approaches to medical investigation. A specific feature of Western culture has been the emphasis on empirically-justified technology and science. The major reason for success has been the development of a consistent set of methodological rules codified in the scientific method. Applied to disease and medicine, this orientation, particularly when combined with a highly involved technology, must inevitably lead to the development of rational and effective medicine. Without such a methodology, the cues available in the external world for the delineation of cause and the discovery of effective treatment are obscured by what I call a "high noise level." This noise level is due to difficulties of diagnosis when internal conditions produce only vague somatic symptoms, and when it is extremely difficult to distinguish one symptom from another. This noise level is increased to crescendo by the fact that most patients get well regardless of therapy. Of course, this noise level can be reduced through carefully structured and controlled experiments, but this is precisely the point where Thai medical systems, in most cases, fall below the mark of the objectivity and empirical orientation required by Western standards.

CONCLUDING REMARKS

In 1981, a campaign was begun to save and revive Thai traditional medicine. As a result, the Foundation for the Promotion of Medicine was established and it planned a new kind of school for traditional doctors, called the College of Ayurvedic Medicine. The philosophy of the school is to prepare graduates to fulfill their duties as medical helpers for the people. As they are well versed in the use of medical technical terms, they are able to work with colleagues in Western medicine. This is in strong contrast to practitioners of older schools of traditional medicine. Very few, if any of them, understand the English medical terminology habitually employed by their Western-trained colleagues.

An attempt is being made to upgrade and integrate Thai and Western medical systems Thai medical practitioners are now required to understand, to a degree, the Western frame of mind. They are trained to use thermometers and stethoscopes in making diagnoses. A synthesis between Western and humoral Thai medicine is certainly desirable. However, is this possible? Consider one problem, that of the relating hot\cold dichotomy--an important part of the diagnostic system in Thai traditional medicine, to the Western biomedical model. How can the "inequilibrium of basic elements" be understood in terms of hypertension, for instance? Could such an integration be achieved even by an expert who knows both Western and Thai medical system very well? I wonder, reasonably so, if there can be any hope of integration. The Thai traditional system of medicine was one of the most effective to have been devised in antiquity. It was more or less closed, as far as its theory went, but it was always open to new ideas for practical therapeutic methods. Thus, Thai traditional medicine has survived to the present and still plays a significant role in Thai medical care. With the support of the government, Thai traditional healers are now trained in a special college where they learn, to some extent, the elements of scientific physiology as well as traditional medicine. Thus they provide an alternative medical service which is effective in the curing of many diseases and is appreciably cheaper than Western medicine. In the process of adapting itself to new conditions, however, the system is losing its personality and is on the way to becoming a poor relation of the modern international system of medicine.

NOTES

1   Aguirre B. *Medicina y Magia*. Mexico, D.F.: Instituto Nacional Indigenista, Coleccion de Antropologia Social, No. 1.
2   Beck B.E.F. Colour and heat in south Indian ritual. *Man*, 4, 1969, 553-572.
3   Chadwick J., and Mann W.N., trans. and eds. *The Medical Works of Hippocrates: A New Translation from the Original Greek*. Blackwell Scientific Publications, 1950.
4   Chuengsatiensap K. Thai medical systems in the rural area. Paper presented at the Thai Traditional Medicine Conference, Bangkok, 1989.
5   Croizier R. *Traditional Medicine in Modern China: Science, Nationalism, and the Tensions of Cultural Change*. Cambridge, Mass: Harvard University Press, 1968.
6   Ketusinh O. A pragmatic modernization of Thai traditional medicine: the College of Ayurvedic Medicine. Lecture delivered at the Institute of Traditional Chinese Medicine, Shanghai, 1982.
7   Ketusinh O. Traditional medicine in Thailand today., Lecture delivered to visiting public health officials from the People's Republic of China, 1982.
8   Laughlin W.S. Primitive theory of medicine: empirical knowledge. In: Galdston I., ed. *Man's Image in Medicine and Anthropology*. New York: International University Press, 1963; 143-152.
9   Pellegrino E.D. Medicine, history, and the idea of man. In: Clausen J.A, Strauss R, eds. *Medicine and Society*. The Annals of the American Academy of Political and Social Science, 1963; 346:9-20.

10   Puntong Gunyarat. Shamanistic healing in Thailand: a preliminary observation. Paper presented at the Conference on Bioethics, Iain Sunan Kaljaga, Yogyakarta, Indonesia December, 18-22, 1989.

11   Rauyajin Oratai and Sam Lee Pliangbangchang. *Psychosocial Aspects of Rural Health Services in the Northern Region of Thailand*. Bangkok: Ministry of Public Health, 1983.

12   Saengvichian Sud. The downfall of Thai traditional medicine and the rising of Western medicine. *Journal of Medical Social Science*, 1978; 1;2: 20-28.

13   Saunders J. *Cultural Difference and Medical Care: The Case of The Spanish-Speaking People of the Southwest*. New York: Russell Sage Foundation, 1954.

14   Torey F.E. *The Mind Game: Witchdoctors and Psychiatrists*. New York: Emerson Hall, 1972.

15   Vajanarat *et al*. *A study of Mon Spirit Dance belief*. Research paper, supported by Mahidol University, 1980.

16   Veith I., trans. *The Yellow Emperor's Classic of Internal Medicine*. Berkeley: University of California Press, 1972.

17   Vibul Polprasert, Suvit, and Komart Chuengsation, eds. *Thai Traditional Medicine Bangkok*: H.N. Press, 1987.

15

Health Policy, Ethics, and Human Values: An International Dialogue

Zbigniew Bankowski

In the fourth book of Plato's *Republic*, Socrates puts the following question to Glaucon: "And the creation of health is the institution of a natural order and government of one by another in the parts of the body? And the creation of disease is the production of a state of things at variance with this natural order?"

For centuries physicians have sought the way, as suggested by the philosopher, to institute a natural order and government in the parts of the body. Not so long ago--indeed within living memory--there was little that medicine could do for the seriously ill, except to offer consolation and some relief from pain. The practice of medicine up to the end of the eighteenth century had hardly advanced since the time of Hippocrates--a period spanning almost two and a half millennia.

In the nineteenth century, means of improving public health were developed, both empirically and scientifically. Great advances in biomedical sciences and health technology, as well as a more profound understanding of the origins and treatment of disease, came only in the present century. Indeed only in recent years has attention begun to be focused on the issues that attend these advances. Ironically, it is these advances that have created new moral and ethical dilemmas in medicine and public health, extending from traditional medical ethics to the new fields of bioethics and health policy ethics.

Faced with the enormous power of medicine for both good and harm, each nation must develop health policies--that is, strategies for optimal use of its health care resources. Many, perhaps most, health policy decisions raise ethical questions. Policies having to do with who shall receive health services, how resources shall be allocated, what criteria should be used in setting priorities, what constitutes acceptable forms of health care, when health care should be begun or ended, even the matter of who should be involved in making policy decisions, all have inherent ethical components. Different national, cultural, and religious traditions yield different ethical value systems, and their interactions with health policymaking will therefore vary from country to country.

Many factors other than ethics influence policy decisions. Political, economic, cultural, religious, and organizational issues can obscure, distort, displace, or promote ethical considerations. Of considerable importance and interest is the dynamics of policymaking, whereby ethical values are taken into account or lost from sight as policies are formulated.

THE ROLE OF ETHICS AND HUMAN VALUES IN HEALTH POLICYMAKING

The ways in which health policy, ethics, and human values interrelate are described by the physician and philosopher, Edmund Pellegrino:

> The *health policy* of a nation or a community is its strategy for controlling and optimizing the social uses of its medical knowledge and resources. Human values are the guides and justifications that people use for choosing the goals, priorities and means that make up that strategy. *Ethics* acts as the bridge between health policy and values. It examines the moral validity of the choices that must be made, and seeks to resolve conflicts between values, which inevitably occur in making those choices. Ethics, therefore, orders human choices in accordance with normative principles.[1]

A health policy, therefore, ultimately reflects the fundamental beliefs and commitments a nation or people ties most closely to its identity and integrity as a human community. These commitments are its human values. Through their expression in the choices and priorities of its health policies a community exerts its influence over the enormous momentum of technological advance. Ethics is itself grounded in sociocultural, philosophical, or religious convictions. These convictions are a society's measuring rods for right and wrong, good and evil. They are often incommensurable and irreconcilable from one culture to another. To examine these convictions or to disagree with them is often perceived as a moral assault because they are so integral to a person's or a nation's self-image.

Health policies are rarely derived from explicit and systematic analysis of the moral values that shape them. Much of the art of national and international politics consists in structuring decisionmaking in such a way that values or issues are *not* confronted. The aim is to keep peace between, and within, divergent belief systems. However, once framed, a health policy unerringly reveals the values that drive a society. This is especially the case in health policies, which so often deal with those in the "shadows" of life--the very young, the poor, the sick, the aged, or the retarded. Different peoples value these groups differently. When resources are limited, tragic choices must be made, which may be to the disadvantage of one group or another.

In every culture there is an unavoidable ethical problem inherent in the very conception of policy formulation. This is the inevitable tension any policy generates between individual and social good. While most policymakers strive to serve both, there is always some point at which further improvements in a society's good intolerably undermines the worthwhileness of each individual's life within that society. According to Pellegrino,[1] three general considerations should motivate health policy and health policymakers:

- First, to attempt to control the social and economic impact of the unrestrained use of advanced medical technology in treating individual patients. The results are now becoming apparent in many countries: prolongation of dying, and increasing the numbers of patients surviving in vegetative states or with lifelong disabilities and handicaps that require large expenditures of human and fiscal resources.
- Second, to achieve a more equitable distribution of the benefits of medical knowledge. What constitutes a "just" principle of distribution will vary from country to country, but each country must confront the issues involved in deciding on some principle of allocation of its resources among health goals, and between health and other social goals.
- Third, to use medical knowledge in an anticipatory way for the collective good of present and future generations. Some examples with very serious moral implications would be policies that would make sterilization or limitation of procreation compulsory for carriers of defective genes; denying life-support measures to defective infants or older patients; manipulating genetic material to control the future physical and behavioral characteristics of the human species along previously determined lines.

Each of the above three purposes arises out of the unprecedented possibilities of modern technology, and each presents some conflict between social and individual good, between traditional medical ethics and social ethics.

Health policy inevitably involves critical choices of ethical and other values, and these, in turn, are drawn from different national and cultural traditions influencing health policy decisionmakers. The influences on those responsible for health policy are diverse--ethical, cultural, political, economic, religious, tribal, bureaucratic, and personal. In any case, the policymaker will make a decision that represents his or her resolution of those diverse influences.

According to Veatch,[2] value systems play at least four different roles:

- First, they provide a framework for choosing among policy alternatives. Policymakers have to consider different feasible options and decide which among them conforms best with the ethical and other values of the group.

- Second, they provide the framework for choosing who the policymakers will be. Choosing the policymakers is to choose the value systems upon which decisions will be made.
- Third, they are critical for deciding which facts will be taken into account and how they will be used for purposes of policymaking.
- Fourth, they are critical in determining what the possibilities are for intercultural cooperation in health policy. There may well be intersection of these cultural traditions that facilitate--indeed require--collaboration across traditions.

It is, therefore, necessary to find out what the basic cultural, ideological, and religious traditions are committed to and what the implications of those commitments are for health policy.

In historical perspective, medicine has been dominated by what could be called the Hippocratic culture. This is the view about medicine that had its beginnings with the Hippocratic writers on the Isle of Cos in ancient Greece and has provided a core of beliefs and values for the medical profession of the Western physician since then. Scholars attribute Hippocratic thought to Pythagoreanism. Important policy judgements were contained in that world view: that the Hippocratic physician should not practice surgery, perform abortions, or give deadly drugs. It also involved a rather unusual division of medicine into three categories: dietetics, pharmacology, and surgery. Hippocratic physicians were encouraged not to take on patients *in extremis*, lest their reputations be hurt. Medical information was viewed as esoteric, too dangerous to make it available to the masses. Modern medical ethics as articulated by professional organizations of physicians remains influenced in varying degrees today by this Hippocratic tradition. Clearly, these philosophical and ethical positions could have considerable impact on anyone responsible for health policy decisions.

It should be equally clear that other philosophies, religions, and secular perspectives and cultural traditions would provide very different ground values for deciding a regional, national, or international health policy. The various traditions often hold well-established views that have great relevance to policy questions about fertility control, care of the chronically ill, allocation of health resources, research on human subjects, and public health.

Even in the more developed West, major cultural and religious traditions often adopt positions that are unique to their own traditions and sometimes incompatible with the Hippocratic tradition. For example, Judaism has serious reservations about autopsy, which the medical community finds critical for gaining further understanding of diseases. Roman Catholics would de-emphasize what they call artificial fertility control, but would be much more tolerant of decisions regarding the terminally ill, letting nature take its course. Still, Western culture, especially in the Anglo-American West, lays an emphasis on individual rights and self-determination that is at odds with the dominant ethos of the medical profession as well as with many other cultural traditions.

The importance of cultural perspective becomes even greater when health policy alternatives are compared across cultures: Hindu views on the relation of this life to future life; Islamic emphasis on the will of Allah; indigenous African views of health and medicine. The central importance of these worldviews-- philosophical, cultural, religious, and political--should not be underestimated as influences on health policy. We are just beginning to understand the significance of these ethical and other values and beliefs. It is unrealistic even to think of resolving these differences; it is not even clear that it would be a good thing to resolve them if we could do so. It is worthwhile, however, to try to understand them, to see how different beliefs, values, and worldviews influence health policy decisions in different cultures.

Some of the differences arise at the most general level. A health policy will be influenced by the extent to which pluralism is central to the ideology of a country--that is, the extent to which it places high value on tolerating and accepting divergent value commitments within its borders. Some countries have an established religion which serves as the source for the ethical and other values that will be incorporated into health policy choices. Others explicitly disavow religious commitments, while others accept religious and nonreligious pluralism in varying degrees.

In addition to the formal ethical systems underlying health policy decisions, it can also be asked how ethical judgments are justified. Are they rooted in rational analysis, in the laws of nature, in religious revelation, or simply in the feelings of particular influential individuals or groups?

Other basic value orientations are reflected in a country's health policy decisions. What is its attitude toward technology? Is it eager to try the newest machinery, committing its health resources to aggressive, high-technology interventions, or is it giving priority to basic or primary health care? To what extent does it feel an obligation to future generations? What is the breadth of its sense of responsibility for health? Does it make policy on the assumption that all members of society should be the beneficiaries of a health policy, or only certain members? Does its responsibility stop at the national borders or is there a belief that national health policy must also take into account the health and welfare of those beyond its borders? Is it a country rooted in a culture oriented to past, present, or future; to conquering nature, living in harmony with it, or being ruled by it?

THE MEANINGS GIVEN TO LIFE, SUFFERING, AND DEATH

Mankind's most fundamental beliefs are those that concern life, suffering, and death--what different societies hold and teach about the origin of man, the purpose of life, the significance of death, and life after death. These beliefs have important implications for health policymaking.

The meanings that *life* holds in different faiths and systems of thought--its origin, the points at which it begins and ends, the degree of control that humans may exercise over its beginning and end, the exact meaning of right to life--cannot be separated from health policymaking.

Health policymakers and professionals are continuously concerned with *suffering*. Whatever their views on its significance and on responses to it, they need to be very sensitive to its significance for those who suffer, and to the religious and cultural determinants of their reactions to it. Both healthcare professionals vis-à-vis their patients and the patients' families, and health policymakers vis-à-vis society, responsible, for instance, for allocating resources for health care, in their own ways have to respond in decisionmaking to the existence of suffering and to its meanings in their societies.

Death means different things to different societies and cultures, and at different times of life. For some it is the end of all life, for others the entrance to another life. In some societies the death of young children is commonplace; in others it is tragic. Whether death should be delayed at all costs is an ethical issue in today's technological societies. The religious significance of death, for individuals and societies, must play a large part in policy decisions about allocating resources for technological means of avoiding death.

We must be concerned with the extent to which the meanings of life, suffering, and death are expressed in the decisions of health policymakers; this is also the extent to which ethical principles govern policymakers' decisions. Assuring social justice and health as a human right may be seen as an objective of society, or the responsibility may be seen as belonging to the individual. When it is seen as the latter, society must assure the conditions in which the individual can exercise this responsibility. In either case, we need to work out explicitly the moral--the ethical--responsibilities of health policymakers who clarify conditions of social justice.

THE CONTRASTS BETWEEN WESTERN AND TRADITIONAL VALUE SYSTEMS

Policymaking logically requires a system of values. Value systems in traditional societies are expressed in forms that differ from those with which Western-trained health professionals are familiar. The ethical formulations that have been worked out in the Western context do not appear to serve well the function of bridging policies and values in traditional societies.

The preoccupation of Western medicine with the organic or materialistic basis of health and illness has led to backwardness in researching and understanding the complex phenomena of complete well-being and disease, and to the alienation of traditional practitioners from the evolution of health policies. It is now evident, for example, that indigenous African healing systems, based on traditional beliefs and medical practices, continue to flourish, and their existence must be taken into account in formulating national health policies.

Secrecy is an essential component of the ethics of many traditional healing systems. Secrecy is expected, for example, to protect society against indiscriminate use of medicines by certain individuals. Secrecy may also have economic implications for native practitioners, in the same way that orthodox "Western" practitioners form associations and regulatory bodies to protect the art and science of healing and to prevent quackery. Excessive secrecy, however, has proved counterproductive in that it has generated suspicion and skepticism about the efficacy of traditional medicine.

In several African societies diseases are believed to be due to either natural or supernatural causes. Of the natural causes, there is little knowledge of micro-organisms, and most communicable diseases are thought to be of supernatural causation; smallpox was a good example. Diseases due to supernatural causes are thought to be induced by human beings by means of sorcery, witchcraft, magic and secret societies, or by divine causes, including the visitation of departed ancestors, angry gods, their earthly priests, or the Almighty. A great deal of traditional medicine is still linked to religion, sympathetic or symbolic magic, and the soul. Nothing seems to happen by itself. Everything is brought about by gods or inflicted by sorcery, witchcraft, or wicked people.

The traditional healer has enormous patience, is part of the community, knows his patients and their ancestors, provides answers to all questions, including how and why, and never admits lack of knowledge; he is aware of the many tensions and conflicts inherent in family and village life. Many Africans, for example, are very stoical in their traditional beliefs about suffering, since it comes from the Almighty or an offended ancestral spirit, or from a wicked sorcerer or witch or some other evil person.

It is apparent that traditional medicine is a comprehensive aggregate of ideas, beliefs, and practices relating not to medicine alone but also to magic, religion, and societal ways of life. It cannot be easily replaced by Western medicine. If its potential for health care is to be realized, developing countries need to make serious efforts to integrate it with the health care delivery system.

Health policymakers, at the international level, need to understand and appreciate the deep origins or sources of human values in different cultures and societies, which always and necessarily underlie health policies. On the basis of such understanding and appreciation we learn to respect one another's beliefs and consequently the different approaches that we take to formulating and implementing health policies.

It is evident that attempts to explore relations between health policies and ethics in an international context carry us beyond the ground where health and ethics are familiar in Western terms, into new territory where cultural values, ideological systems, and even the meanings given to societal development appear in different and often puzzling forms. New questions appear that can be answered only in cross-cultural dialogue, and dialogue leads us, of necessity, toward a profoundly deeper understanding of one another.

Neither health policymakers, health care professionals, nor ethicists can explore such issues effectively alone: true transdisciplinarity is required. To provide a forum for an international, intercultural dialogue for the improvement of the understanding of relationships between health policy-making, ethics, and human values in different cultural settings, the Council for International

Organization of Medical Sciences (CIOMS) initiated in 1985 a program entitled "Health Policy, Ethics, and Human Values--An International Dialogue." This International Dialogue includes in its objectives the development of transcultural and transdisciplinary approaches and methods in this field and the use of improved understanding of approaches of various societies to the ethical and human values aspects of health policy as a way to pursue deeper human understanding of human values across cultural and political lines.

The main means of implementing the program is the organization of international, intercultural conferences with a global orientation, or regional conferences concerned with the interaction of health policymaking, ethics, and human values in culturally, largely homogeneous settings.

As examples of regional conferences, in 1986 in New Delhi, a conference, organized in the framework of the dialogue, considered the interaction of health policymaking, ethics, and human values from an Indian perspective; in 1987 at Noordwijk in the Netherlands, from a European and North American perspective; and in 1988 in Cairo, from an Islamic perspective.

An example of a globally-oriented conference was that held in 1988 in Bangkok, on "Ethics and Human Values in Family Planning," which considered the ethical issues inherent in family planning from different national and cultural perspectives.

Another example is the conference on "Genetics, Ethics, and Human Values: Human Genome Mapping, Genetic Screening, and Genetic Therapy," to be held in 1990 in Japan. It is aimed at stimulating an international, interdisciplinary, and transcultural dialogue on the ethical implications of research in molecular genetics, particularly those of mapping and sequencing the human genome.

When we consider the world in all its diversity, it is strongly apparent that we need to achieve a common basis for policy transcending the viewpoints of each particular group. Of course, we must respect all that is deeply important to people, and this certainly includes their religious convictions, whatever they are. We can agree that dogmatism, fanaticism, and ideology are the enemies of tolerance, of careful listening, of reason, and of understanding and compassion for those who are different. They foster divisiveness and conflict, and the health of the people of the world is far too important for us to accept that. Instead, we should turn our efforts to identifying that core of principles on which we can agree, and should strive to have them adopted as a basis of an *international code of ethics for health policy*. We must live with the reality of disagreement about some issues, but we should do all we can to translate our considerable agreement into better health for mankind.

NOTES

1   Pellegrino E.D. Keynote address: Health policy, ethics and human values. In: Bankowski Z., Bryant J.H., eds. *Health Policy, Ethics and Human Values--An*

International Dialogue. Geneva: Council for International Organizations of Medical Sciences, 1985;7-17.

2   Veatch R. "Value systems: their roles in shaping policy decisions." In: Bankowski Z., Bryant J.H., eds. Health Policy, Ethics and Human Values--An International Dialogue. Geneva: Council for International Organizations of Medical Sciences, 1985;84-86.